THE REAL DOCTOR WILL SEE YOU SHORTLY

ALSO BY MATT MCCARTHY

Odd Man Out: A Year on the Mound with a Minor League Misfit

THE REAL DOCTOR WILL SEE YOU SHORTLY

A Physician's First Year

—•—

MATT McCARTHY

CROWN PUBLISHERS
NEW YORK

Copyright © 2015 by Matt McCarthy

Published in the United States by Crown Publishers, an imprint of the Crown Publishing Group, a division of Penguin Random House LLC, New York.
www.crownpublishing.com

CROWN is a registered trademark and the Crown colophon is a trademark of Penguin Random House LLC.

Library of Congress Cataloging-in-Publication Data
McCarthy, Matt.
  The real doctor will see you shortly : a physician's first year / by Matt McCarthy.
    pages cm
  1. McCarthy, Matt. 2. Medical students—New York (State)—New York—Biography.
3. Interns (Medicine)—New York (State)—New York—Biography. 4. Residents
(Medicine)—New York (State)—New York—Biography. I. Title.
  R154.M156A3 2015
  610.71'55092—dc23
  [B]

                                                                    2014037870

ISBN 978-0-8041-3865-9
eBook ISBN 978-0-8041-3866-6

Printed in the United States of America

Jacket design by Ben Wiseman
Jacket photograph by Johanna Parkin/Getty Images

10 9 8 7 6 5 4 3 2 1

First Edition

For Heather

Author's Note

This is a true story and the people I've written about are real. However, in order to ensure patient privacy and maintain the confidentiality of others, this work has been carefully vetted to comply with the Health Insurance Portability and Accountability Act (HIPAA), and throughout the book, names, dates, and personal identifying details have been changed. In one instance, a composite character has been used.

Prologue

It started with a banana peel.

After years of quiet study in the libraries, laboratories, and lecture halls of Harvard Medical School, I finally made the tectonic shift to hospital life in the summer of 2006. The third year of medical school marks a startling departure from the academic fantasia of study groups and pass/fail exams, and I was flooded with anxiety. I valued sleep. I wasn't sure how I'd handle destructive criticism, and I was known to have an irritable bowel.

The first assignment in my rotation was surgery, a three-month slog of 120-hour workweeks at Massachusetts General Hospital that was designed to identify the handful of future surgeons in our class of roughly 165 students. On the first day, I was assigned to a team with a desiccated fifth-year surgical resident named Axel, who had piercing periwinkle eyes and an implausible Adam's apple that caused my eyes to bounce when he spoke. Axel could fairly be described as a member of the Undead; he had traded the better part of his youth for world-class surgical training and wasn't sure it had been a fair swap.

Shortly after I was introduced to him in the cafeteria, Axel held up a banana peel, tore it in half, and said, "You may not lay a hand on any of my patients until you've sutured this back together." He reached in his back pocket, handed me a needle and thread, and banished me from sight. "Go wherever you want to figure it out," he said, "and please stop grinding your teeth."

At first I didn't know what to do; surely none of the other medical students had been given this assignment, and I didn't know my way around the place we called Man's Greatest Hospital well enough to find someone who could help. I cradled the peel like a wounded bird and started wandering up and down the long corridors, peeking into rooms at random. Eventually I returned to the room where I'd started the day—the surgical library—where an administrative assistant had given a dozen of us folders with an outline of expectations. There had been no mention of banana peels.

As I scanned the room, which was dotted with portraits of men I should have recognized but didn't, I recalled something a frustrated professor had recently said to me: "When a patient is having a heart attack, a Harvard student's instinct is to sprint not to the patient's bedside but rather to the library, to read more about the nature of chest pain. Don't ever do that." Yet here I was, surrounded by books instead of patients.

I pulled one off the shelf and flipped through the pages. What were my classmates doing right now? Learning to scrub in? Assisting with appendectomies? Removing gallbladders? That's what I'd thought this rotation would be about: actual surgery, not fumbling with fruit. Was all of that really on hold until I figured this out? I looked down at the banana peel and sighed.

I could probably patch the thing back together with some basic shoestring knots, but that wasn't the task. Suturing involves a specific set of techniques to make knots that leave very little trace of their existence, as would be necessary on a patient who required them to close up a wound. But the instructions I found in books weren't helping. The pages were filled with detailed descriptions of arcane anatomical structures and artists' renderings of complex intestinal surgeries, stuff that was far too advanced for me.

Based on my incipient attempts, the banana peel would have been grounds for a malpractice suit. An olio of solutions bounced through my head: *Pay a frazzled surgical intern to show me how to suture? Superglue the peel back together? Claim I'd used dissolving stitches?*

I heard a knock at the door and closed the book. A voice outside the library called, "Hey, a little help?"

I opened the door and found looking up at me a man with a receding hairline and wire-rimmed glasses seated in a wheelchair.

"Hello," I said, as though receiving an uninvited dinner guest. A lost patient, I presumed, until the man wheeled himself past me into the room and flipped on a second set of lights. "I'm Charlie," he said. "You must be . . ."

"Matt. One of the new medical students."

His face brightened, and he took off the glasses. "Charlie McCabe," he said. "Pleasure to meet you."

I flinched when I heard the name. McCabe had been one of the most promising surgeons of his generation when he began his residency at Mass General in the 1970s. At the end of his training, he was accepted into the cardiothoracic subspecialty training program at MGH, but just before graduation, he developed a tingling in his hands. In short measure he was diagnosed with multiple sclerosis and was left unable to operate. After the diagnosis, McCabe began teaching surgery to medical students and now ran the surgical rotation at Mass General. He had been named the Harvard Medical School teacher of the year on several occasions, and we all knew his heartbreaking biography.

"You're a few minutes early," he said. "I was about to have you guys paged. We're going to go over some of the basics of the rotation."

As I sat down I looked for a place to put the peel.

"Need a trash can?" McCabe asked, motioning with his head toward the large receptacle in the corner.

"My, uh, resident gave this to me today to—"

"Axel and his banana peels." McCabe's head shook from side to side.

"Yes."

"Give it a shot, and if you can't figure it out I'll show you."

"Really?"

"Give it a shot."

———

For the next three days, I reported to the surgical library at 6:00 A.M. to spend hour upon frustrating hour mutilating the ever-darkening, softening banana peel. At the end of the third day, I bumped into McCabe near the hospital's entrance.

"Success?" he asked. I held up the tattered peel, and he winced and said, "To my office."

When we got to his office, I took a seat and he handed me a suture kit that he kept on his desk. "Technique is crucial," he said. "Are you right-handed or left?"

"Left."

"Southpaw!" he said. "All right."

The last time I'd been called that was on a baseball diamond, when life had seemed to be pulling me in a very different direction. Before I met McCabe, I'd spent four years on the Yale baseball team, day-dreaming of life as a professional athlete. A week after graduation, I was drafted in the twenty-first round of the 2002 Major League Base-ball draft by the Anaheim Angels and joined a minor-league team in Provo, Utah.

It quickly became apparent, however, that our hero was not destined for a career in pro ball. And it was during that soul-searching summer in the minors that I acknowledged something my sister had said during our childhood in Florida: I was one of the very few athletes who just didn't look good in a baseball cap. So as my brief but memorable stint in rookie ball drew to a close, I applied to medical school. Harvard accepted me the same month I was cut by the Angels.

McCabe's hands shook as he positioned mine above the banana peel and approximated its edges. The sensation made me shiver, which I tried not to show; he seemed as delicate as the peel. But despite the shaking he moved with remarkable certainty. His confidence and ex-pertise were undiminished, and I could imagine in that moment how good he must've been. "Don't take too big of a bite," McCabe said, referring to the depth of the needle insertion. "But be confident, be assertive."

I made a swipe, and he shook his head. "Not bad. Not good. Again." I retracted the needle and considered my next path. "You're thinking," he said. "Don't think. Do." I took another swipe, and the peel cinched together. "Perfect." I was briefly reminded of the pottery-throwing scene from *Ghost*. What felt clumsy at first quickly became comfortable. The peel was sutured up in minutes. "You're a natural," he said. "I think we might have a budding surgeon on our hands."

The compliment stilled my roiling stomach. To have picked up something so quickly gave me a hint of the confidence I'd felt in baseball, before I peaked short of the big leagues and suddenly started hearing from coaches and trainers that I didn't quite have what it took. Granted, I had a long way to go in medical school, but this sort of stroking coming from someone like McCabe opened up a window on a possible future.

I admired the dank, battered peel and presented it to Axel the next morning over a predawn breakfast. "Very nice," he said, daintily holding the peel over his plate of pancakes. "You're almost ready for the show."

As I took in the compliment, I thought about the operating room and "the show." I imagined myself extracting a bullet from a victim of senseless violence and calmly suturing up the wound.

"Let's lay some ground rules." Axel mumbled while devouring his food. "One, you should always be the first one scrubbed in. Two, do not speak unless spoken to. Three, wear a clean pair of scrubs every day and keep a shirt and tie in your locker for the days when we have clinic."

"Got it." I started to write *TIE* on my hand.

"Please do not write on your hands."

We got up from our pancakes, and when Axel discarded his tray and the beat-up banana peel, I realized with a twinge of sadness that

I'd grown somewhat fond of it. As we headed toward the operating room, he put his right hand on my left shoulder and stopped me. He was tall but wiry, not imposing.

"Going to give you some words of wisdom," he said, "that were passed down to me when I became a surgeon. Consider them a surgeon's survival guide." I closed my eyes briefly, indicating I was ready to absorb. "When you can eat, eat. When you can sleep, sleep. When you can fuck, fuck. But do not fuck with the pancreas."

With the banana peel successfully sutured, Axel assigned me a mélange of increasingly complex tasks. I was invited into the operating room and allowed to navigate the laparoscope while he removed diseased organs, and before long I was the one excising the appendix or gallbladder (but not the pancreas, of course). Medical school, it seemed, was like baseball or the arts: neophytes showing aptitude received more attention from instructors and were put in better positions to succeed.

In the Massachusetts General emergency room, I learned to suture human skin. My first patients were a series of unconscious victims of motor vehicle accidents in need of a few arm or leg stitches, and I thrilled at watching open wounds close neatly at the pull of a thread. From there I moved to conscious patients, and soon I was stitching faces. As the terror in my patients' eyes gave way, so did mine. The first facial laceration I dealt with was on a woman who'd been bitten in the lip by her pet toucan. Axel emphasized the importance of lining up her lip properly before throwing the first stitch.

"If the vermilion border is misaligned," he said, manipulating her lips, "she'll be permanently disfigured. Now, go to it."

Sewing people up soon revealed itself as a sophisticated craft, or perhaps art, to which I could devote myself. It presented a focused canvas full of microdecisions, but there was always an optimal solution to any surgical question—the correct way to align the sides of a wound, the best place to throw the first stitch. One could see how surgeons with aptitude gained mastery through repetition, how they could joke about performing certain surgeries in their sleep.

I found the process of putting someone back together deeply affecting. Day after day, I scoured the waiting room looking for lacerations, and any chance to further hone my skills. I sensed that my role as promising student affected Axel, too. He seemed less hollowed-out, less vehement, and he dispensed nuggets of wisdom with increasing frequency:

"Don't wear a bow tie to work before you're forty. Makes you look like a douche bag."
"Trauma surgeons don't worry about follow-up appointments."
"Don't shit where you eat."
"Don't buy a motorcycle."

At the end of the three-month rotation, Charlie McCabe called me into his office. As I removed the suture kit from my back pocket so I could sit down, we both looked at the spot on his desk where he'd first shown me how to use a needle and thread. McCabe took off his glasses and clumsily cleaned them with a handkerchief.

"I'm going to cut to the chase," he said. "You've got talent. I've talked to Axel, I've spoken to my colleagues. I've seen it with my own eyes." I fought back a smile. "Personally, I think you'd be crazy to do anything other than spend the rest of your life in the operating room." I had been raised Catholic, and though I had stopped going to church sometime in college, McCabe's words sprinkled down on me like holy water from an aspergillum. "But I'm not gonna bullshit you," he went on. "It's hard. At this stage you need to ask yourself a very basic and deceptively simple question: Can I imagine myself being happy as anything other than a surgeon?"

By this point I had a great deal invested in making Charlie Mc-Cabe happy. But sitting across from him at age twenty-six, I knew the answer to his question was probably yes. I'd never considered life as a surgeon until a few weeks ago, and while I enjoyed the work—it was new, it was thrilling—I wasn't convinced that surgery was my calling. I could handle waking up at 4:15 A.M. now, but what about when I was forty? Or (gasp) fifty? None of the surgeons I knew actually seemed happy. But who does?

Axel was someone I admired, but not someone I envied. The few times I overheard him on his phone, he was breaking plans, not making them. The brusque manner and bags under his eyes gave me a small window into his difficult, stressful life, and I wasn't sure it was for me.

"I enjoy being in the operating room," I said haltingly. McCabe was a man who had trained some of the country's best surgeons. I didn't want to blow a life-changing opportunity, but I also didn't want to be dishonest with him or myself. I was going to blow it. "Can I get back to you?" I asked.

McCabe looked down at his desk and smiled the way one might in mixed company at an off-color joke. "Sure," he said softly. "Of course."

Those skills I learned in surgery—suturing, navigating a laparoscope, clipping a wayward artery—were my fondest memories of medical school. I possessed an intricate, highly specialized skill set, but it was of no use to me, two weeks removed from my Harvard Medical School graduation in June 2008, as I prepared to face my first night on call in Columbia University Medical Center's cardiac care unit.

PART I

I

Carl Gladstone woke on the west side of Manhattan in the small hours of June 18, 2008. The professor, as was his custom, put on a pot of coffee and loped into the shower. After trimming his mustache and inspecting his thinning brown mane, he may have revisited a question that had been nagging him. Did he, in fact, look like Theodore Roosevelt, as one of his students had recently suggested?

Gladstone grabbed his briefcase and Yankees baseball cap and headed out of the Hell's Kitchen apartment to his office. A northbound train ride deposited him at a college in Westchester County, where he'd spent the entirety of his academic career, teaching accounting. After catching up on email, scanning the Yankees box score, and perhaps agonizing over the one thing that could possibly drive him to an early retirement—deriving new questions for his exams—he stood up, tucked in his shirt, and walked down the hall to an empty classroom.

As the students filed in for the 11:00 A.M. class, Gladstone methodically began to write on a chalkboard. Satisfied with his work, he pivoted to survey the room. He cleared his throat to call the chattering students to order. Then he felt a twinge in his right arm.

A moment later, he was on the floor.

Quick-thinking students dropped their backpacks and phones and lunged into action; an ambulance was called, and despite momentary doubts ("Do we really give our teacher mouth-to-mouth?"), a young man initiated CPR. After several awkward attempts at chest compressions, Gladstone regained consciousness as quickly as he had lost it. He stood up, backed away from the students, and asked everyone to return to their seats.

Within minutes, an ambulance arrived. After some haggling with the emergency medical technicians, Gladstone acknowledged that he was still having chest pain and agreed to be transported to the Columbia University Medical Center. As the ambulance took off, emergency room physicians and nurses received notification of Gladstone's impending arrival. By the time his stretcher burst through the swinging doors of the ER, a cardiologist was waiting for him.

Nurses instantly slapped twelve EKG leads on his chest as the team transferred him from the ambulance stretcher to an emergency cot. Gladstone was surely unaware of the unusual EKG report the leads were generating just a few feet from his head. The report, which resembled a red-and-white checkered seismograph, was retrieved by the bedside cardiologist. It revealed broad, irregular waves that plateaued rather than forming sharp points, a finding known as tombstoning because of its grave prognostic implications. A large segment of his heart had suddenly and unexpectedly lost blood flow.

Seeing the tombstones, the cardiologist informed the emergency room staff that there was no time for X-rays or blood tests. Gladstone was rushed upstairs and into a dark room—the cardiac catheterization lab—where a team of interventional cardiologists went to work on his convulsing, failing heart. Gasping for air, Gladstone was quickly sedated and a large tube called a cardiac catheter was plunged into his groin, then snaked into his aorta. A doctor shot dye through the catheter and into his heart's blood vessels, and the image was projected onto a flat-screen monitor for the team to see. There were a few silent nods as the image became clear. His left main coronary artery was blocked—an abnormality known as the widow maker's lesion—and the cardiologists quickly went about opening it up by inflating and deflating a small balloon that rested on a guide wire at the end of the catheter.

Time to treatment is critical; restoration of blood flow in the obstructed artery is the key determinant of both short- and long-term outcomes for patients suffering heart attacks. Hospitals are now evaluated by the time that elapses from a patient's arrival in the emergency room until the balloon has been inflated inside the clogged artery. This door-to-balloon time should be no more than ninety minutes according to the American Heart Association. For Carl Gladstone, it had been less than fifty.

After the senior interventional cardiologist deemed the procedure a success, a still-sedated Gladstone was placed on yet another stretcher and transported to the cardiac care unit, an eighteen-bed intensive care unit on the fifth floor of the hospital for cardiac patients requiring continuous monitoring. Dr. Gladstone would live to see another day, but he would not be able to appreciate the statistical misfortune of being placed in the care of a physician who had been practicing medicine for less than a week, a physician who could not yet interpret a subtle but potentially devastating clinical finding.

Me.

2

Seeing a new patient wheeled into the cardiac care unit, I leapt up from my seat.

"Easy," said the physician next to me. He placed a hand on my shoulder and guided me back into my chair like a trainer gentling an unsteady colt. "Give the nurses a few minutes to do their thing." He spoke softly and bore a surprising resemblance to a *Charles in Charge*– era Scott Baio, all black hair and good-natured smiles. His nose was perhaps slightly too small for his face, in contrast to mine, of which the reverse was true. "The nurses are going to do a lot more for him tonight than you and I are."

I nodded and eased back into my seat. "Okay," I said to Baio as I straightened my scrub top. I was anxious. I was excited. I'd just chugged a large iced coffee and could hardly sit still.

After my surgery experience with Axel and McCabe, I had moved on to Harvard's rotations in neurology, psychiatry, radiology, internal medicine, pediatrics, and finally, obstetrics, where a young Jamaican woman let me deliver her child on my first day. She insisted on giving birth on her hands and knees, her back arched like that of a cat as the baby slowly emerged. An amused midwife later said that I had looked like a nervous quarterback, receiving a snap in slow motion.

As medical school graduation approached, choosing a specialty had proved to be difficult. Ultimately I had settled on internal medicine because it was the broadest field, the one that might allow me to feel like a jack-of-all-trades. But tonight was my debut in the big show, a thirty-hour shift taking care of critically ill patients and responding effectively to anyone who might roll through the door.

"We've got a few minutes," Baio continued, "and I know this is your first night in the hospital. So let's go over a few things."

"Great!" I replied. Our orientation leaders, a peppy group of second- and third-year residents, had instructed us to exude a demented degree of enthusiasm at all times, which wasn't difficult now that my blood was more caffeine than hemoglobin.

"Just relax," he said, "and take a look around."

Together we scanned the fluorescent room, an enclosed space the size of a tennis court containing critically ill patients and upwardly mobile Filipino nurses bustling between them. The perimeter, painted a regrettable shade of yellow, housed the patients in glass cubicles, while the center, where we were sitting, was mission control, filled with chairs, tables, and computers.

"It's just you and me tonight," Baio said, whipping his stethoscope back and forth around his neck. "And eighteen of the sickest patients in the hospital."

Every night an intern and a second-year resident presided over the CCU. Tonight was our turn, as it would be every fourth night for the next month. All of the patients in the unit were on ventilators except one, a large Hispanic man who was riding a stationary bicycle and watching *Judge Judy* in his room. "These patients are receiving some of the most complex and sophisticated therapies in the world." Baio reached for an antebellum bagel that was sitting on a platter nearby. "Patients get referred to the cardiac care unit when hope is lost or after something devastating happens. Balloon pumps, ventricular assist devices, transplanted hearts, you name it."

Until a few days ago, I had never set foot in a cardiac care unit. Nothing about the setup looked terribly familiar. I continued to study the room, trying to decode the symphony of incessant beeps and alarms and wondering what each of them meant. It felt like I was sitting in the middle of a giant equation with infinite variables.

"These patients should all be dead," Baio went on. "Almost every one of them is kept alive by an artificial method. And every day they're going to try to die on us. But we're going to keep them alive." He paused for effect. "And that's fucking cool."

It was fucking cool. Back before my stint in the minors, I had studied molecular biophysics and briefly flirted with the idea of going to graduate school in that subject, using my degree to solve the structure of molecules that were too small to be seen under a microscope. But the field lost me when a professor, a young crystallographer, introduced the importance of imaginary numbers in biophysics. Try as I might, I just couldn't wrap my head around that quixotic concept. I wanted to translate science into something more concrete, more tactile, to seek a profession where I could touch and see and feel. So I changed course and pursued medicine. And thus far, it had seemed like a wise decision. Nothing about this moment with Baio seemed imaginary. Quite the contrary, it felt excessively real.

Baio wiped off the bagel crumbs on his scrubs and leaned in close to me, bringing scores of punctate pores on his nose into focus. "We have to work as a team. Everything is teamwork. So I need to know what you're able to do. The more you can do, the more time I have to think about the patients. So rather than listing the shit you can't do, tell me what you can do."

My mind went blank. Or more accurately, I searched it and found it was blank. "Well . . ." I glanced at the sedated patient before us. He was on a ventilator and had a half dozen tubes in his neck, arms, and groin, almost all of which pulsed with medications I'd never heard of. As a medical student, I had been exposed to all sorts of patients. But all of those encounters had involved walking, talking, reasonably well-functioning individuals. Lying there, inert and blanched of all color, the patient before me seemed well beyond the reach of my limited powers. If he needed his appendix out or his face stitched together, I was his man. But intensive cardiac care? The learning curve in medicine was so unforgivably steep. What could I possibly do to assist him?

Finally Baio broke the silence. "All right," he said, "I'll start. Can you draw blood?"

"No."

"Can you put in an IV?"

"No."

"Can you put in a nasogastric tube?"

"I can try."

"Ha. That's a no. Ever done a paracentesis?"

"I'd love to learn."

He smiled. "Did you actually go to medical school?"

Even I had to wonder. If Baio had been asking me to recite pages from a journal article on kidney chemistry or coagulation cascades, I could've put on quite a show. But I hadn't learned much of the practical business of keeping people alive, skills like drawing blood or putting in a urinary catheter. Harvard hadn't prioritized them. In fact I had been allowed to skip the CCU month of my med school training at Mass General so I could learn tropical medicine in Indonesia. Who had talked me into that?

"I graduated from Harvard earlier this month."

"Oh, I know you went to Haaahvaahd," Baio said with exaggerated fake reverence. "But do you know how to order medications?"

A bright spot. "Some!" I practically beamed.

"Do you know how to write a note?"

"Yes." The moment I said it I realized just how paltry a contribution it would seem to him. Baio must have seen my face drop.

"That will actually be a big help," he said. "Examine every patient and write a note on them for the chart. That will save me time. You need to be concise yet precise."

I grabbed my small notebook and scribbled *examine everyone/write notes.*

"And listen," he said while chewing on the stale bagel, "if I want a sandwich tonight, go to the cafeteria to get me a sandwich. And if I ask for a coffee when you return and give me that sandwich, do you know what you should do?"

"Head to Starbucks."

"Correct."

One of the nurses tapped me on the shoulder and asked me to order a blood thinner for a patient, but Baio cut her off. "Dr. McCarthy is not yet a functioning member of society," he told her before putting in the order himself. I watched over his shoulder as he typed away.

"The nurses will know what medication the patient needs before you do," Baio said.

"I've heard that."

After finishing with the order, Baio turned and looked me up and down while grabbing another bagel. "You may be thinking, Why is this guy an asshole?"

I shook my head. "I'm not. I wasn't."

"Well, I'm not an asshole." He returned to the computer. "I'm stuck in this enclosed unit for the next twenty-something hours. I can't leave. The only way I can step outside of this unit is if a cardiac arrest is called over the intercom and I have to go bring someone back to life."

"Got it."

"And if that happens, you're alone in here. It's just you. All alone. And them," he said, spinning his hand once around his head.

Jesus.

"Now, if you keep me well fed and caffeinated, I will be happy. And if I'm happy, I will feel inspired to teach you a thing or two about how to actually be a doctor."

And that was the truth of it. Baio, one year my senior, would essentially be teaching me how to be a physician. It was hard to believe he had been an intern just last week; the man looked like a sample photo at Supercuts. At Columbia, as at most teaching hospitals, interns were paired with second-year residents to manage between twelve and eighteen patients, and were provided with varying levels of supervision by attending, board-certified physicians who met with us every morning at 7:30 to discuss our plans for the day. But the guts of the day, the minute-to-minute, I'd spend hooked to Baio.

"I want nothing more than to keep these patients alive," I offered, perhaps a touch too earnestly.

He waved his hand at me. "Yeah, yeah. Just show up on time and bust your ass." This I could do. It was a philosophy a former baseball coach of mine had sworn by. "Looking at you, I'm thinking two things," Baio said. "One, you kinda look like someone I know. You both look like big ol' meatballs."

It was not the first time my admittedly WASP jock appearance had been skewered by a member of the healthcare community. In medical school, a female classmate named Heather had told me without prompting that I looked like my name was Chad and I attended prep school in Connecticut. This woman, who bore more than a passing resemblance to Anna Chlumsky from *My Girl,* would be surprised to learn that I'd spent the first decade of my life in Birmingham, Alabama, and the second in the indeterminate sprawl of a suburb outside of Orlando, Florida. I'd won her over after accepting a dare to ask a well-regarded diabetes researcher if he'd ever considered calling the condition "live-abetes" to give it a more positive spin. He was not amused. But she was; we'd started dating shortly thereafter and had come to New York together to join Columbia's internal medicine training program. Heather was in her second year of residency, a year ahead of me. I wished she were here to whisper advice into my ear.

"What's the other thing?" I asked Baio.

He smiled. "You look terrified."

"I am."

"Good. Go examine our new patient."

3

"Still asleep," the nurse said as I drew back the curtain and poked my head into one of the partitioned glass cubes on the unit's perimeter. "He's all yours."

Behind the nurse, the room's windows opened onto the Hudson River, but the view was obscured by a mountain of medical equipment. In the center of the room a male patient lay sedated in a large bed with guardrails that had been ergonomically designed to prevent bedsores. If too much pressure was applied to one side, sensors would activate and the mattress would inflate to balance the force. Behind the bed stood what appeared to be a stainless-steel coatrack upon which hung nine different plastic bags filled with clear fluid, each about the size of a breast implant. Above these, monitors slightly larger than an iPhone screen displayed the names of the medications in the bags and the rate at which they were being administered. If a bag became empty, an alarm would sound. If someone tampered with the rate, a whistle would blow. The whole setup looked like a cryptic art installation of sirens, machines, buttons, tubes, wires, and blinking lights. I had been given very clear instructions during orientation: aside from the patient, don't touch anything in the room.

I took a deep breath and approached the unconscious patient, a mustachioed man who looked a bit like Teddy Roosevelt. I grabbed a pair of gloves and prepared to examine this mysterious man who had been dropped into our laps by whatever fate had befallen him. I thought back to medical school and how I was taught to perform a physical examination.

"Start with the hands," my instructor had advised. "It will put the patient at ease and will reveal how a person lives, how they eat, how they work, if they smoke . . ."

I put on the gloves and picked up the man's limp right hand. It looked like a normal hand, pink and soft, and without dirt under the nails. No evidence of the small hemorrhages known as Janeway lesions or the lumps known as Osler's nodes, named for physicians of a bygone era and each indicative of an infected heart valve. From the hand I moved up the arm, looking for track marks—signs of IV drug use, which could also predispose the heart to infection. From there I shifted my attention to his head, where I noted a small abrasion on his scalp. Throughout my examination, his chest gently oscillated up and down as the ventilator forced half a liter of air into his lungs every five seconds.

"Mr. Gladstone," I said.

No response. I was almost relieved, but then I remembered another nugget of medical school wisdom. "You do not want to be the physician who assumed the patient was sleeping," the instructor had told us, "when in fact he was dead."

"Mr. Gladstone!" I shouted, too loud.

The patient let out a soft whimper. I moved to his eyes, lifting each lid up with my left hand while using my right to shine a penlight in; both pupils contracted as they should. I waved my finger toward his nose, assessing the ability to focus on a near object, a process called accommodation. His pupils, which easily reacted to light, could not accommodate. Before moving on to the nose, I noted that the left pupil appeared two millimeters smaller than the right.

As I jotted my findings in a small notepad, the ambient noise of the unit faded into the background. It was just the two of us alone in a vacuum. I raised my eyes from my notes and stared at the patient's chest, watching it quietly heave with every manufactured breath. What was his heart doing under there? Was he recovering or dying? "You're going to get through this," I whispered, more to myself than to him. I wondered where Carl Gladstone was from and how he spent his days. Did he work? Did he have a family?

ARREST STAT, SIX GARDEN SOUTH! the intercom blared overhead. *ARREST STAT, SIX GARDEN SOUTH!*

I turned away from the patient to see Baio sprinting past the room, grinning, a man utterly in his element. "It's just you, bud!" he said as he pushed the unit doors open. "Hold down the fort!"

And with that, I was alone in the unit, the doors swinging gently on their springed hinges in Baio's wake. I closed my eyes and cursed under my breath. Quickly completing my examination of Carl Gladstone, I typed up a note to reflect my findings. With every sentence, I looked around the room, certain that someone's heart had stopped. I was alone, and filled with an electrifying sense of nowness.

Baio returned after twenty agonizingly long minutes.

"How'd it go?" I asked.

"Just saved a life," he said, smiling. His jockish pride reminded me of former teammates and my former life. "How is our new patient?"

"Wow, that's great. What happened?"

"Priorities, my friend. Tell me about our new patient first."

"Sure, sure," I answered, pulling up my notes. "Fifty-eight-year-old guy had a heart attack. Kinda random. Just went to work, teaching a class, and dropped to the floor."

"Not random," Baio said flatly.

I paused, recalling our conversation on rounds a day earlier. Baio had mentioned that cardiovascular functions are influenced by circadian rhythms, and as a result, heart attacks are much more common in the morning hours.

"Right."

"Go on," Baio said. "You have my undivided attention."

"They took him to the cath lab and fixed him."

His eyes locked onto mine and he wrinkled his brow. "And that's it?"

"He's a little sleepy right now, but yeah, that's it."

"Anything else you'd like to tell me?"

"I think that's the big picture. On exam he looks pretty good. Still sedated but stable. I'm sure there's more detail in here," I said, reaching for his chart.

Baio grabbed the cranberry chart before I could and shook his head in frustration. "You have told me almost no useful information."

I scratched my chin, avoiding eye contact. I hated to disappoint this man. I wanted to be like him. I wanted to *be* him. "One pupil is smaller than the other," I offered.

Baio looked up. "Well, that *is* interesting. What do you make of it? What's your differential diagnosis?" he asked, referring to the systematic process of elimination in which a clinician considers an array of maladies before arriving at a diagnosis. This was how I had been taught to approach any symptom or clinical finding in medical school. The cause of something simple—a cough, for example—could ultimately be so obscure that we were encouraged to initially think as broadly as possible. This expansive list, which was quickly pared down, was known as the differential diagnosis. Our professors at Harvard had routinely amazed us with the inconceivably long lists they could generate.

I had been pleased with myself for noting the unequal pupils but hadn't really taken the next step and considered the cause. I was the dial-up to Baio's broadband, the MySpace to his Twitter. I thought back to a mnemonic I'd been taught in medical school to generate a differential diagnosis: VINDICATE.

V—Vascular

"He could be having a stroke," I said. "Maybe there's a vascular process in his brain causing one pupil to constrict."

I—Infection

"He could have an infection of the pupil—something like herpes of the eyeball."

N—Neoplasm

"He could have a neoplastic process—a tumor of the eye or brain cancer."

D—Drugs

"He received a number of painkillers in the ambulance and a sedative before the catheterization. I know narcotics can affect the pupils."

Baio touched his index finger to my chest, almost sweetly. "I'm impressed."

"Thank you," I said, fighting back a smile.

"Now, it's great to rattle off a bunch of possible causes, but what are we actually putting our money on?"

Medical school was for generating a list, I thought. But being a doctor means knowing how to narrow that list. "Well," I said as my eyes quickly moved back and forth, "I doubt it's cancer, might be a stroke. Less likely infection. It's probably the drugs."

"Sounds reasonable," Baio said, closing the chart. "Listen, we need to work on your presentations. I need to know about these patients in far greater detail than you just gave me."

"Okay." I reached for my notebook and quickly jotted down *details!*

"But first let me tell you about that cardiac arrest."

"Yeah, that's right. What happened?"

"Whenever I run to an arrest, I whisper 'ABC, ABC' to remind myself that it's got to start with airway, breathing, circulation."

I scribbled *ABC.*

"Don't write this down, just listen," he said. "So I get into the room and this dude isn't moving. His eyes are open but nobody's home. Not responding to anything. So imagine you're me. What do you do?"

The thought paralyzed me. "I have no idea."

"That is not the right answer, Dr. McCarthy. Think."

"Let's see . . ."

"But remember, in real time you don't have the luxury of thinking about it."

"It has to be instinctual," I said awkwardly.

"What did you say to yourself while sprinting?"

"ABC . . ." A hint of a smile from Baio. "So," I went on. "A . . . airway. I would assess the airway."

"Bingo."

"Did the patient have an open airway?"

"I checked his airway and it was blocked. So we intubated him on the spot."

"Nice."

"And when the tube went into his throat, all this shit came out."

Baio removed his white coat, displaying innumerable smudges on his scrub top.

"What do you think it was?" I asked.

"Oh, it was shit. Actual feces."

I put my hand over my mouth. Holding on to his undershirt with his right hand, Baio pulled the scrub top off with his left and bundled it into a ball.

"But how could—"

Before I could finish the thought, the scrub top hit me in the face.

"We'll talk more about it later," he said, as he sauntered away to examine Carl Gladstone. "Go introduce yourself to the rest of our guests."

4

Looking for a patient with whom I could interact, I elected to begin with the only one who was ambulatory: the large man on the stationary bike.

"Hello," I said, gently tapping on the glass divider separating the patient's room from the rest of the unit. He stopped pedaling and took off his headphones. A Hispanic man in his early forties, he had a shaved head and a room littered with books, magazines, and scraps of handwritten notes. He was stocky, barrel-chested, and broad-shouldered like an ex-linebacker, and by the looks of things he had been in the unit for quite some time.

"Hi," I continued as I entered the room, "I'm . . ."

"One of the new guys."

"Yes."

"Benny Santos," he said, extending a hand. "It's a pleasure." He spoke softly and deliberately and had a surprisingly smooth hand. Unlike the other patients, he was not in a hospital gown. Instead, he wore a New York Giants T-shirt and jeans.

"I'm one of the new physicians here," I said, avoiding the word *intern*.

"Welcome."

Catching sight of a notebook by his bed, I paused and tried to figure out how to ask this rather large, well-appearing man why he was in a critical care unit.

"Why am I here? . . . Is that what you're wondering?" he said, flashing a smile. His voice was so soft that I found myself leaning in close to catch his words.

"It is."

"Need a new ticker," he said, pointing at his chest.

Outside his room, we overheard a senior physician giving an evening tour to a group of medical students. "Many of the patients in this unit," the guide said, "are among the more than five million Americans living with heart failure—a condition in which the heart is unable to pump sufficient blood to the body."

"That's me," Benny said cheerfully, "star attraction."

"Failing to deliver blood to starving organs," the guide continued, "fluid gradually backs up into the lungs as the kidneys and liver inevitably fail. At that point, no medication or dietary modification can save them. It's transplant or bust."

"Been here for several months," Benny said softly, "just waiting."

I thought of how I'd spent the past few weeks—graduation parties, move to Manhattan, orientation cocktails. "That's tough," I offered. On the other hand, his relatively stable condition meant one less patient for me to worry about.

"Just trying to sneak up the UNOS list," he said. On rounds as a medical student I had been introduced to the United Network for Organ Sharing and its sophisticated algorithm for allocating organs; it varied significantly by city, but the median wait time for a new heart was expected to be just over 150 days. Benny, however, was on his way to becoming an unfortunate outlier.

"What are you listening to?" I asked. This was a mistake. I wanted to make a connection, but discussing music was a huge weak spot for me. In college I'd once been laughed out of a dorm room for saying that I felt like the Goo Goo Dolls were playing the sound track to my life.

"A little Babyface," he said. "You a fan?"

"I can't say that I am."

"Okay, okay. That's cool."

"Judge Judy, on the other hand," I added, motioning toward the television, "huge fan."

He smiled, and we looked up at the television. "Yeah, she's great. Very wise."

My teeth grinding came to a halt and I took a seat on the edge of his bed. "They call her the White Oprah," I said.

Benny wrinkled his brow as Judy banged her gavel. "Who calls her that?"

"Didn't someone call her that?"

"I don't think so," he said. "Definitely not."

Benny looked out of the window, onto the Henry Hudson Parkway, where traffic was backed up for miles. "I really appreciate you guys coming in here, checking on me periodically, shooting the shit and whatnot."

"Of course."

"You know, one of your colleagues used to come in here, spent fifteen or twenty minutes with me every single day. Talk about Scripture, talk about music, anything."

"That's great."

"One day we were both here on a holiday. I was down, and she could tell I wasn't my normal, charming self. So we're looking out the window just like this and she says, you know, more traffic accidents happen on holidays. Drunk drivers, more people on the roads, stuff like that."

I nodded.

"And she smiles and says, 'Every drunk driver, every family coming back from the beach . . . those could be organ donors.' Every crash brings me closer to a transplant."

He turned from the window and looked at me.

I wasn't sure what reaction was called for here. "I suppose that's one way of looking at it," I responded.

He frowned. "That's a horrible way of looking at it!"

"Yes, that is a horrible way of looking at it."

I blushed, embarrassed by the exchange.

"She meant well," he said, glancing up with a smile, "but no one would mistake your colleague for White Oprah."

5

"New patient looks okay," Baio said of Gladstone a few minutes later as he grabbed two chairs and led me to the back of the unit. "His wife is coming in shortly. Needs to wake up a bit, so I stopped the sedatives."

"Got it, I'll put in the order."

"I already took care of it. Okay, let's play a game."

Our last conversation had ended with a shit-stained scrub top landing in my face; I shuddered to think how a "game" could turn out.

"A year from now, you're going to be in charge of running a cardiac arrest. Dozens of doctors, crammed in a room, looking at you while a lifeless patient lies in the middle. This year you get off easy—you just do chest compressions or draw blood or put in an IV. But next year you're the conductor."

"Fantastic," I deadpanned. Running a cardiac arrest was not a scenario that had been covered much in medical school. And perhaps with good reason—the mere thought of it would have given many of us nightmares. We had been more focused on learning and perfecting the basics of listening to patients and examining them.

"I'm going to throw scenarios at you and I want you to tell me how you'd handle them. Ready?"

I laughed. "I think we both know the answer is no. But . . . yes."

"Okay, it's six A.M., you show up for work and start checking on your patients. You enter a room and the patient is unresponsive. Twenty-four-year-old black girl. Go."

He pointed at me, and I slowly exhaled. Beeping ventilators and vital signs monitors were momentarily ignored. "Unresponsive?"

"Unconscious, unresponsive. Whatever. She doesn't move when you shake her. Go."

"I suppose . . . I suppose I'd start with the ABCs."

"Fine. She has a patent airway, but she's not breathing and her heart's not beating."

I smiled, trying to buy time. "We should fix that." My mind was in overdrive, desperately trying to draw on the events of the one cardiac arrest I'd witnessed at Massachusetts General.

"Indeed."

"I would intubate her," I said, "and start chest compressions."

"Good, and can you do both of those things?"

"No. Not at the same time."

"So . . ." he said, jutting his chin forward.

"I'd get help. I'd yell for help."

"Excellent!" Baio patted my arm. "In this case, your inclination to react like a small child is correct. Everything in medicine is based around teamwork. Never forget that. So, what else?"

"I'm not sure."

"You've started CPR, you're giving her oxygen. But why would a young girl's heart stop?" His green eyes narrowed slightly, focusing on me intently.

It shouldn't, I thought. "Congenital something or other?" I offered.

"I said she was a twenty-something black girl. Does that help?"

"Maybe she overdosed?"

"Easy"—he laughed, leaning away from me—"not all black kids are on drugs."

I was aghast. "No, no, no, I just—"

"I'm kidding—drugs are a reasonable thought. What would you do about it?"

"I could give something maybe to reverse the drugs."

"Yes. Narcan. It's incredible. Turns someone from a stuporous zombie to agitated and annoying in seconds. What if I told you she had a fistula on her arm?"

"She could have a kidney disease."

"Go on . . ."

"Maybe she missed dialysis or maybe her electrolytes are off. I'd ask someone to draw labs. Maybe the potassium . . ."

He shook his head. "The woman's heart isn't beating. Do you have any idea how long it would take our lab to process her blood and tell us about the potassium?"

"No."

"She'd be in the morgue before you had your answer."

I rubbed my forehead. "Shit." I had reached for the textbook again and the patient was dead. So when was I supposed to reach for the textbook? How could I know what to do if I didn't know what to do?

"You have to be one step ahead," said Baio. "Treat empirically. Assume her potassium is off and treat it. You have to be comfortable flying blind. And please stop grinding your teeth."

"I'm trying."

"Let's do another. You enter the room, and this time it's a banker that's unresponsive."

"What kind of banker?"

"I don't know," he said, waving his hand, "a banker. Shuffles paper around, makes a lot of money. A banker."

"Let's see," I said, looking at the ceiling, "could be . . . cocaine?"

"Everyone's on drugs with you," he said, smiling, as he reached for a small carton of apple juice. "I like it. Keep going."

As he took a large sip, a nurse sprinted in our direction. Her heavy footfall broke my concentration, and we both looked up as she reached us.

"It's Ms. Franklin!" she said.

Baio stood up and reactively tugged on my sleeve. "Let's do this," he said, beaming, and started to sprint down the hallway. I followed him as quickly as I could. As we ran, he said over his shoulder, "Do everything I say. Everything."

We quickly arrived at the bedside of an elderly woman on a ventilator. She was so frail and thin that you could make out the individual muscle fibers in her neck.

"What happened?" Baio asked a nurse standing at the bedside. Before she could answer, Baio turned to me. "Matt, disconnect her from the ventilator."

A team of nurses went to work on the woman. "She just flatlined," one of them said.

I looked at the breathing machine and my stomach turned. I suddenly had an overwhelming urge to move my bowels. Disconnecting a patient from a ventilator was a scenario I had only read about in medical ethics textbooks. Terri Schiavo came to mind.

"Disconnect," Baio repeated calmly while reaching a hand under her gown and onto her groin, searching for a pulse.

I tugged the breathing tube away from the ventilator, but nothing happened. I tried again but still nothing. A nurse half my size lunged in front of me and pulled the breathing tube off of the ventilator in one quick motion as Baio rattled off a series of questions while assigning each nurse a specific role in the resuscitation. Someone began squeezing a bag of oxygen into her throat as I rapidly glanced back and forth at the flurry of activity, looking for something to do. Baio briefly closed his eyes while again feeling under the gown. "No pulse. Matt, start chest compressions."

I positioned myself on the left side of the bed and placed one hand over the other. I had performed CPR dozens of times on Janet, the Mass General crash test dummy, but never on a human before. A moment of terror shot through me as I pondered the implications of my 190-pound body descending upon this 87-pound woman.

Baio sensed my hesitation. "Just accept that you're going to break her ribs. Just do it. She's dead. Let's go."

With the first thrust, ribs cracked as easily as uncooked spaghetti.

"Aah," I muttered. With my second compression, more ribs cracked. By the third compression, her chest cavity had become soft and I could feel the sharp edges of broken ribs under her skin.

To the nurse beside him, Baio said, "I will need one round of epinephrine and one round of atropine." Placing his hands in sterile gloves, he reached for a large needle and again mashed on her groin, searching for a pulse. "Slow down, Matt, you're pumping too fast. One hundred beats a minute."

He began to insert a large tube into her pelvis.

"Staying alive," he said.

"Yeah, she is . . ." I said, becoming short of breath.

"No, she is dead. But the song 'Stayin' Alive,' remember? Do compressions to that beat."

I didn't remember because I'd been in the restroom earlier that day while the team discussed that chest compressions should be performed roughly one hundred times per minute. In the heat of the moment, it's nearly impossible to keep track of the pace, but the Bee Gees' song "Stayin' Alive," which happens to play at 103 beats per minute, could be used to help keep the pace.

"Stop chest compressions," Baio said firmly.

I stopped and caught my breath. The patient's chest was sunken where I'd been pounding away. We looked at the defibrillator monitor. I desperately wanted to do something else, anything. I was not ready to see the second patient I'd touched die in front of me after I cracked her body open performing chest compressions.

"The monitor shows a heartbeat," I said between breaths.

Baio placed his hand on her neck. "No pulse. Resume compressions."

The heartbeat I'd seen was not really a heartbeat, rather something called pulseless electrical activity. Her heart was spasming as electrical currents raced across cell walls; to the inexperienced eye (mine) it would appear like beats on a heart monitor. But without a pulse there was not sufficient blood flow to the body. Baio was right: CPR had to continue.

I resumed my assault on her chest cavity as a nurse injected one medication after another into her. The sharp edges of her broken ribs felt like they were about to slice through her skin.

Baio kept his eyes trained on the monitor. "Hold compressions, and Matt, feel for a pulse."

I placed my hand on her neck and felt nothing. My heart sank. "I don't—"

Baio simultaneously felt the other side.

"Oh, yep"—he smiled—"there's a pulse. Congratulations. You just saved your first life."

He moved my hand several inches higher, where indeed, there was a vigorous, bounding pulse.

"Holy shit!" I said as we locked eyes.

"Holy shit, indeed. Now, put her back on the ventilator."

This was it. After years of preparation, I had just helped bring someone back from the dead. My heart raced, and I could feel my own pulse pounding through my neck. This was the sensation I had been seeking, the one that was missing for me in surgery. Granted, I had done exactly what Baio told me to do, and it had involved damaging the patient in ways that seemed to create a new set of problems, but she had pulled through. She was stayin' alive, and would live to see another day with her spouse, kids, whomever. Medicine was messy, but it was fucking incredible. As we stood together at the bedside, I looked over at Baio with a measure of pride. He seemed to sense this.

"You know," he said, patting me on the back, "there is nothing more rewarding than bringing a ninety-five-year-old demented woman with widely metastatic lung cancer back to life. Well done."

6

I spent the next few hours peering over Baio's shoulder as he put out one fire after another. It was like being in the front row of a small concert, mesmerized by an undiscovered band on the cusp of stardom, thinking, Why didn't I ever learn to play the guitar? On each of my trips to the cafeteria to retrieve snacks, I filled my notebook with terms and phrases to look up. It was three in the morning before I knew it, and twenty-one hours of my shift had elapsed in the blink of an eye.

Or had it? I had seen and done more in this one night than I had in entire months of medical school. A beating heart had stopped and I'd restarted it with the thumps of my palms. I'd broken ribs, mashed on groins, adjusted ventilators, and administered medications that were so new they didn't appear in textbooks. Sure it was fun to delicately suture a facial laceration, but there was something unique, something otherworldly about critical care medicine. The patients were so sick, so close to death; there were no imaginary numbers in the cardiac care unit. The operating room seemed almost mundane by comparison. Axel would surely laugh at the suggestion, but he was missing out. Surgery had come to seem narrow to me; this was complex decision making that involved processing dozens of inputs at once.

Back at the nurses' station, Baio emphatically struck a letter on the keyboard and spun in my direction. "All right, I'm wired and I'm happy. Time for some teaching. Let's go over some EKGs. I will assume you are absolutely horrible at reading these," he said, fighting back a smile.

I grabbed my pen and wheeled my chair closer to him. "That is an excellent assumption."

"Let's start with your new patient, Gladstone," he said, holding up the EKG that hours earlier had set so many wheels in motion. "Everything we do in medicine has to be systematic."

Systematic, I said to myself, ready to make it a mantra.

"Otherwise, things get missed and bad shit happens."

"Understood."

"When I look at an EKG, I say the same thing to myself every time: rate, rhythm, axis, interval. I start with the rate. Do you know why I start there?"

I shook my head.

"If the rate is wildly abnormal—say a hundred and ninety beats per minute . . . or twenty-five beats per minute—you need to drop the EKG and go evaluate the patient. Got it?"

I scribbled, *wildly abnormal rate, drop ekg.* "Yes, yes. Got it. Consider it a brain tattoo."

"You remind me"—he chuckled—"you remind me a little bit of that dude from *Memento.*"

I considered the movie's handsome star for a moment and said, "Thanks."

"Not a compliment. Next, I examine rhythm. If the rhythm is anything other than normal sinus rhythm, we could have an issue."

Over the next two and a half hours, Baio showed me how to read an EKG, interpret an arterial blood gas report, and process the deluge of data that was generated on each patient every few hours. I wished I'd been doing this from day one of medical school. Countless anatomy or pharmacology lectures had armed me with volumes of critical information and yet no way to translate it into the actual practice of being a doctor. Dealing with life-or-death situations required knowing not just body chemistry and physical science but how to assess a patient's condition correctly and make quick decisions. And without a framework for organizing all the knowledge in my head for quick application, I was certain to flounder. What Baio was doing in the CCU, I realized, was providing a way of merging the knowledge in my head with the reality of my patients' symptoms.

Around 5:30 A.M., physicians, including my three cointerns, began to file into the CCU. I had been assigned at random to spend the entirety of my three-year residency training with the same three women: Ariel, Lalitha, and Meghan. We would take turns working thirty-hour shifts every fourth day for the majority of the year. But our time together was somewhat limited in the CCU because we'd each been paired up with second-year physicians—in my case Baio—to learn the ropes. Every four weeks for the entire year, the four of us would move to a new rotation—infectious diseases, general medicine, geriatrics, medical intensive care, oncology, et cetera. In our second year, we would repeat the cycle while supervising an intern each, essentially becoming Baio, an idea that was mercifully remote. I couldn't quite tell you what third-year residents did, other than apply for jobs or subspecialty fellowships.

"Breakfast!" Ariel said, handing me a brown paper bag and a coffee. She had frizzy red hair and green designer scrubs with a blue racing stripe.

Baio grabbed the bag and examined its contents. Dissatisfied with the options, he looked up. "How is your pod?" he asked, which was what the hospital called each team of interns.

"They seem nice. Great, actually."

"Better hope you get along. You don't see much of them now, but you will. You've got eighty hours a week, every week, for the next three years."

"Hard to believe."

"Personality conflicts," he said with a mischievous grin, "can make for a bumpy ride."

The interpersonal dynamics of working closely with three other interns for three years in a high-stakes environment were not yet clear to me. But it appeared that these trial-by-fire friendships would emerge in small bursts, and would be based wholly on trust. If my colleagues couldn't rely on me, if they couldn't be sure that I would take care of their patients as well as they could, our group would be dysfunctional. No amount of kindness or humor or empathy could overcome that. Without a shared sense of trust, we would have nothing.

I spent the next hour reviewing my patients and preparing for rounds. At 7:00 A.M. a new set of nurses arrived.

"Give them some space," Baio said. "Let's talk."

I walked with him to a corner of the unit.

"Our attending is going to be here soon," he said, referring to the board-certified cardiologist supervising us all. "He's a total badass. Cardiologist to the stars. He's brilliant but tough. Doesn't like his time to be wasted. So make your presentations short. Get to the point. Tell him what he needs to know about the patient and move on. Got it?"

Thirty minutes later, rounds started. Eleven of us gathered in a white-coat-clad horseshoe around Dr. Badass: four interns, four residents, a medical student, a pharmacist, and a cardiology fellow named Diego, who was originally from Argentina. Diego had completed his residency training at Columbia and was now in the prestigious three-year cardiology fellowship, learning to become the Badass much like I was learning to become Baio. He had a perpetual squint and reminded me of Axel when I first met him—tired, curt, and wholly unimpressed with me.

Our group stood in silence, waiting for the Badass to speak. I had been up for twenty-six hours, and delirium was setting in. At twelve hours, I had been tired. At sixteen, a second wind had kicked in. But by twenty-four hours, basic faculties started failing, and now I felt about three hours away from needing to be admitted myself. The endurance marathon of the thirty-hour shift confused me. How could I be responsible for my patients if I was in worse shape than they were?

Slowly, heads turned in my direction and the Badass said, "Well?"

Baio nudged me and whispered, "You're on, dude."

It has been said that if you look around a poker table and can't immediately spot the sucker, it's you. I feared I might now be in the midst of something similar. I squeezed my notes and brought them up to my face. The word *Gladstone* popped out along with *anisocoria,* and in a margin, I had apparently scrawled *solo synchronized swimming—an Olympic sport?,* something I didn't remember writing.

"Carl Gladstone is a fifty-eight-year-old man with no significant past medical history who developed chest pain at work yesterday," I began, reading from my notes. "Collapsed and was brought to our ER."

I had everyone's attention, with the exception of Baio, who was whispering in a nurse's ear. When I was finished, we entered the room and collectively examined my patient. I spoke for a few minutes more as Diego stared at the tile floor, gently shaking his head, before the Badass interrupted.

"Fine. Next patient. The thing about the pupil is strange. Scan his head."

Bleary-eyed and stammering away, I proceeded to present the events of each patient as we moved around the unit. Most of it I got right, some of it I got wrong. Fortunately, my well-rested team was there to step in if I misinterpreted an EKG finding or misstated a lab value. As we approached Benny's room, the Badass softly said, "Next," and we continued past. Mercifully, I was dismissed after rounds and asked Baio if he wanted to head to the subway with me.

"Nah," he said, "I'm gonna stick around for a bit." He picked up a stack of EKGs and yawned. "By the way, nice work last night."

With the gait of someone about to fail a sobriety test, I walked to the elevator and out of the hospital into the warm summer sun. It was just after noon and I had been awake for more than thirty hours—a new personal best. Crossing the street, I saw a large red banner draped down the side of a hospital overpass.

Amazing Things Are Happening Here!

The words made me smile. How could I possibly describe the things I'd just seen and done? *Amazing* seemed as good an adjective as any. A few minutes later I plopped into an empty seat on a southbound subway car and drifted off to sleep.

7

I was back in the unit the next day before sunrise. Benny waved from his bike each time I passed his window, hustling from one room to the next, familiarizing myself with the new patients. A woman was now residing in Gladstone's recently vacated bed. He had been transferred to another floor shortly before his wife, Sasha, arrived searching for answers. I gave her my best summary of the situation but ultimately referred her to my supervisor for a complete explanation. On her way out of the unit, she flagged me down to express her gratitude.

"He's going to get through this," I said, hoping that my optimistic spin on the situation was appropriate and, more important, accurate. It was a good sign that he was no longer in the unit, but I really couldn't speak to his long-term prognosis. Sasha, with hair so white it appeared to be dyed, was twisting her lip back and forth as we spoke.

"I pray you're right," she said.

I grabbed her right hand and gave it a soft squeeze. "We have to stay positive."

"Did you get to talk with him at all?"

"I did not."

"He's one of those creatures of habit. Starts every day the same." She repositioned her purse on her shoulder and smiled at the thought of her husband's routine. "Makes coffee, hops in the shower. Goes to his office. I don't understand why the other day was different."

"We're going to do everything in our power to answer that." Her lip quivered as I spoke. "Tell me more about him," I said.

A few minutes later, Baio, standing in front of a chest X-ray, summoned me. "We're going to do at least five minutes of teaching every day. Today's lesson is the chest X-ray."

I grinned. "That's very kind of you."

"I'm not doing it out of kindness. I'm doing it so you're not a terrible doctor." He slapped me on the back and grinned. "Okay, how do you read a chest X-ray?"

"Systematically," I said, thinking about his approach to any- and everything.

"Correct. Without a system, things get missed. So what's your system?"

"I don't really . . . I know I should, but I don't have one. I just kinda look at it. Like here," I said, pointing at a white blot in the left lung, "pneumonia."

"No!" He shook his head. "You've got to be better than that. But at least you're honest. Take another stab at it."

If Baio was Charles in charge, I was Charles's dopey pal on the show, Buddy Lembeck. Perhaps it wasn't pneumonia, but it certainly looked like it. "Okay, the left lung appears to show pneumonia and the right lung . . ."

"Stop."

"What?"

"If you see a beautiful woman on the street," he said earnestly, "do you first look at her chest?"

I wondered if this was a trick question.

"The answer is no, Dr. McCarthy. Start in the periphery. Does she have an ankle tattoo? Or a wedding ring? Then work your way in."

I nodded. "Okay."

"If you went straight for the lungs, you'd miss this at the edge."

He pointed at a hairline fracture of the left clavicle. He was right: I certainly would've missed it.

"Let's get started," Dr. Badass bellowed from the other end of the hallway. "Chop, chop. Cut the bullshit."

Rounds began promptly at 7:30 A.M. and proceeded at a dizzying pace. Blips of conversation were exchanged between the more senior members of the group in a medical shorthand that I was not yet able to fully process. My role was to present the overnight events on a handful of patients and to give a short presentation based on a question I had asked on rounds a day earlier, when I wondered aloud how long we had been doing heart transplants at Columbia. As it turned out, if you posed a question on rounds for which there was not an immediate and obvious answer, you would be asked to give a short presentation on the subject the following day.

In between presentations, I occasionally whispered questions to Baio, searching for further explanation of an acronym or clinical trial, but each time he held an index finger to his lips and shook his head. My notebook continued to fill up throughout the morning. We finished rounds shortly before noon. As I jotted down *cardioversion,* I felt a hand on my shoulder. It was the Badass.

"You're doing a nice job," he said softly, his large brown eyes staring down at me. It was the first time we'd spoken outside of rounds, and thus far I'd found him as approachable as a supermodel. Innumerable wrinkles lined his forehead and cheeks, and his hair looked like wet hay. "But, Dr. McCarthy, you should really know how to read a damn chest X-ray."

After lunch, a ninety-second affair in which we gobbled down gamey tuna fish sandwiches, Baio gave me the task of placing a large-bore IV, what's known as a central line, into the femoral vein of a young woman. Baio would supervise the procedure and suggested I watch a simulation of it on *The New England Journal of Medicine* website.

Shortly after the video began, someone tapped me on the shoulder.

"Phone call for you, Doc," said the ward clerk.

I paused the video simulation and took the phone, wondering who knew to reach me in the unit. "Dr. McCarthy?" said the man.

"Speaking."

"This is Dr. Sothscott." He had a soft baritone and spoke quickly. Residents and attending physicians often called the CCU in search of an explanation or clarification pertaining to a patient recently transferred out of our unit, but they never asked to speak to me.

"Hi," I said tentatively.

"I'll cut to the chase," he said, "you took care of a Carl Gladstone."

"Yes. Are you—"

"I am."

"How is he? I noticed he left the unit."

"Well, I'll get to that," he said before blowing a deep breath into the phone. "I'm sitting here reading your note on him and I want to commend you on your thorough physical examination."

A pleasant surprise.

"You performed an exhaustive ocular exam and correctly spotted anisocoria."

The different sizes of his pupils. "Thank you."

"Let me continue. Your note goes on to attribute this pupillary asymmetry to the sedatives he received."

"Yes."

"Now, Dr. McCarthy," he said, his voice rising slightly, "what medication did you attribute it to . . . specifically?"

I scanned my memory. Images of the handwritten notes in his chart fluttered across my brain. "Hmm. Well, he received several sedatives."

"He did indeed."

"I'll have to admit I don't remember all of the medications he received."

"No problem," he replied. "I have a list right in front of me. I'll read them to you."

A medical variation of the Socratic method, I suspected, as he went through the list. It was a little annoying. I already had one Baio.

"I . . . I think several of them can cause pupillary constriction," I offered.

"Right again." There was a pause, and I looked at Baio, who was revolving his fingers to indicate that I should wrap up the conversation. It was time for me to insert the large IV.

"But how many, Dr. McCarthy, cause unilateral pupillary constriction of the kind you observed?"

I thought for a moment, suddenly wondering if I was speaking with another resident or an attending. "Off the top of my head . . ." I said.

"Oh, Doctor, this need not be off the top of your head." His speech was becoming urgent. "Please, use references. Use a textbook. Use the Internet. Phone a friend. But please tell me, in all of medical literature, has anyone ever identified an intravenous medication that shrinks one pupil but not the other?"

Another pause. Now I wasn't sure.

"The answer is no!" he screamed.

My head shot back from the phone.

"Carl Gladstone was on a blood thinner for a clot in his leg. When he fell and hit his head in his classroom," Sothscott continued, barely able to contain himself, "he started bleeding in his brain."

I closed my eyes.

"And I know you know he fell because you documented the abrasion on his scalp."

"Oh . . . no," I said softly and turned away from Baio.

"Oh, yes. And when you saw him, Dr. McCarthy, the blood was flooding his brain and starting to impinge on his cranial nerves."

I couldn't breathe.

"Yet your note does not reflect that. Your note is completely misleading. And it does a shocking disservice to—"

"I . . ."

"How much time was wasted?" he demanded.

"I am so sorry." I wanted to hide. I wanted to disappear. I wanted to run, but there was nowhere to go. I was terrified to think of what I had done to Carl Gladstone. It had been more than a day since the Badass had said to scan his head. Was he bleeding the whole time until he reached Sothscott? That kind of time could have killed him. My knees buckled and I crouched toward the tiled floor, gasping for air as my eyes welled up.

8

The conversation with Sothscott left me hollow, paralyzed. I closed my eyes, tracing and retracing the creases in my palms as I tried to make sense of it. I had just told Carl Gladstone's wife that he was going to be okay, that he'd get through this, all as I had almost single-handedly assured that this would not be the case. I dug my fingernails deep into my hands, creating a physical discomfort that served as a blissful, vivifying moment of distraction from the perverse mixture of worry, fear, and anxiety. I opened my eyes and again examined the creases. They almost formed letters—an *A* in my left palm and an *M* in my right. I searched for significance but drew a blank. Then I felt a tap on the shoulder.

"What is this?" Baio asked. "What's happening?" Trying to compose myself, I looked up. Did Baio already know about the error? Did Dr. Badass? "Are some amazing things happening here?"

"Well." Part of me wanted to blurt out the entire conversation with Sothscott. But a bigger part didn't. Baio wasn't responsible for leaving notes on patients; that was the intern's job. There was no documentation of his faulty reasoning, only my own. I felt like I was going to throw up.

"Are you okay?" he asked.

"Not really."

"You look terrible."

"I'm not feeling well." I didn't know where to begin. "I'll be back in a minute," I murmured.

I went to the only place of refuge I could think of—the call room, with its lilac walls, buzzing fluorescent lights, and flimsy bunk beds. It would almost certainly be deserted at this time of day. I punched in the three-digit code and headed for the bathroom. Catching a brief image of my face in the mirror—I looked like wet shit—I bit my bottom lip and dry-heaved over the toilet bowl.

My arms went limp as my face turned into a damp mess. But I had to get back to the CCU. In the room next to Benny's, there was a young woman in need of the large-bore IV. I threw cold water on my face and tried to focus on her story so I could momentarily forget about my own. Her name was Denise Lundquist, and she had just been transferred to us from a hospital in New Jersey. Baio had obtained her medical records and explained to me that a few days earlier, she had come home from work to find her husband, Peter, in the kitchen, holding his head in his hands. Peter informed Denise that her brother had been killed in a traffic accident. Upon hearing this, Denise collapsed; minutes later an ambulance arrived and took her to a local hospital, where it was revealed that she, like Gladstone, had suffered a massive heart attack.

It was a terrible story, but the details were a welcome distraction. After a seemingly successful catheterization, Denise's heart had continued to deteriorate as her lungs filled with fluid. Doctors ultimately placed her on a respirator, at which point they also made the decision to transfer her to our CCU, which was better equipped to deal with such critically ill, unstable patients.

I grabbed a paper towel and dabbed my face. I had to get back to work. Denise needed the large IV to receive a cocktail of potentially lifesaving medications, and every second I spent in the call room delayed her treatment. When I reentered the CCU a minute later, Baio had already started the procedure. By the time I had put on my gloves and disposable gown, the IV had been inserted.

"Go home, dude," Baio said as he walked out of the room. "Come back when you're ready to work."

I shook my head, remembering some of the first words he ever said to me: *We have to work as a team. Everything is teamwork.*

"Seriously," he said, glancing around the unit. "Go. There's not much left to do today. Go."

After a weak protest, I was on the southbound 1 train to my apartment, wondering how my absence might affect the others. What would they think? Exiting at Seventy-Ninth Street, I blew past my large Eastern Bloc doorman with a small wave before he could get a word out. Heather was still at work, seeing patients in her primary care clinic. I had the apartment to myself. I dropped my shoulder bag and spilled its contents—stethoscope, white coat, and a small bible called *Pocket Medicine*—on my living room floor, collapsed on the couch, and slept soundly through the night.

I woke the next morning to the caterwauls of small children outside my window, and immediately my anxiety came flooding back. How was I going to face the day? I had no emotional frame of reference for something like this. Something so grave, so awful. A swirl of questions bombarded my conscience. What had happened to Carl Gladstone after he left the unit? What would I say to Baio? Should I just keep the phone call to myself and move on? And was that even possible? If someone found out, were we in danger of being sued? I imagined for a moment having to tell people that I'd been a doctor for two days but then I accidentally killed someone. The thought made me almost throw up again.

I pulled an outfit out of my closet and took a deep breath as I recalled a small silver lining: my schedule today would take me out of the cardiac care unit in the afternoon, down to the other end of 168th Street to begin work in a primary care clinic. As part of my medical training, I also had to learn how to treat everyday complaints like back pain or the sniffles. Many residents found the transition to a slower pace more difficult; they included Baio, who warned that primary care would be the most painful part of my medical education. Other residents loved it, considering it a much-needed change from the frantic pace of the hospital. Given what I'd just been through in the CCU, an afternoon spent in an office chatting with patients who were in no immediate danger of dying seemed like a godsend.

As the subway lurched northward into the dewy morning, I overheard two young men considering Barack Obama's chances in the upcoming election—both agreed he had promise but was ultimately too inexperienced—and my thoughts turned inward to my own inexperience. My medical school diploma hadn't yet been framed and already I found myself racked with guilt.

On the other hand, it seemed impossible that this was all my fault. I had told Baio my differential diagnosis on the anisocoria, but he didn't have to listen to me. He could make his own clinical decisions. His job was to show *me* the ropes. What the hell did I know? One might say this was really a case of faulty oversight. Still, I felt like shit trying to blame Baio, and either way it didn't change what happened to Carl Gladstone. Or maybe Baio hadn't listened to me; maybe he'd called my sedative suggestion "reasonable" but ultimately ignored it. What if I wrote a note that didn't reflect what actually happened to my patient? I was very confused.

My mind continued to wander, as it often did on the subway. Were these first few days in the hospital a sign of things to come or just a bump in the road? People enter medical school with the belief that they're on the path to becoming revered, trustworthy physicians, but what if I was destined to become the one colleagues whispered about? Maybe it would be safer to have me tucked away in a laboratory, tinkering with those imaginary numbers and—

"Excuse me, ladies and gentlemen!" a man in the center of the subway shouted. "It is your lucky day!"

I looked up to see a black man a few steps away dressed in a purple bathrobe and sandals.

"My name is Ali and I am an internationally renowned spiritual healer."

I pulled out *Heart Disease for Dummies*.

"I have been blessed with the clairvoyant powers of my ancestral spirit and I am here to help you!"

Ali looked up and down the aisle, largely ignored, and raised his tawny arms. His facial hair had been fashioned into a Vandyke beard, and I guessed he was originally from West Africa. "My powers include, but are not limited to: bringing back loved ones, depression, substance abuse, debt, and impotence!"

The woman next to me put down her *New York Times* and looked up at him.

"I can also help with court cases, immigration status, breaking black magic, breaking curses, breaking jinxes, and all general demonic forces that may cause you trouble!"

He paced the length of the subway car, tying and untying the bathrobe. "Your pain is my responsibility," he continued. "I can also help with success in business, success in sports, and SAT prep!"

He produced a stack of cream-colored business cards from the bathrobe pockets and handed one to me. It read:

ALI

YOU KNOW I CAN HELP

YOU KNOW WHERE TO FIND ME

I put down the book and stared at the card. I wasn't a superstitious person, but at the moment I was willing to indulge almost any fantasy that my life could be improved instantly. Was this some sort of sign? After all, I did need help. I was unprepared for the extremes of emotion that medicine provided and found myself in search of something—a moral compass, a mood stabilizer—anything to get me through the ups and downs of hospital life. What if Ali was actually some font of wisdom who could provide sage if unexpected advice to guide me through my career?

As I rubbed the business card between my thumb and forefinger, wondering how Heather would react if I asked if Ali could move in with us, the neighboring passenger tapped my knee with her newspaper. "Last week," she whispered, "this guy was selling candy for youth basketball."

9

After another haphazard morning spent collecting and interpreting laboratory and physical exam findings in the cardiac care unit, Baio pulled me aside. I braced for what was coming.

"We should talk," he said. I made a point to look him in the eye, but he largely avoided meeting my gaze. This was unusual. Baio was a man who could process an astounding array of information and immediately make sense of it all; he must have known what happened with Gladstone.

"Yeah," I said, bracing for an accusation or explanation. But he said nothing, so I did. "When I saw the pupil—"

"Your presentations are weak," he said. "Pick it up."

A wave of relief. "I've sensed that."

"Here's the key," he said, glancing at his pager. "You've only got a few minutes before we lose interest. Every word has to count."

Being on safe conversational ground was simultaneously relieving and nerve-racking. Wasn't I just delaying the inevitable? Wasn't the first rule of public relations to get out ahead of the story? I couldn't do it. The longer we avoided discussing it, the worse I felt. Why wasn't he saying anything? He probably realized we were both culpable. But what about Diego or the Badass?

"Your presentation has to be problem-based," he went on. "Why is the person in the unit and what are the barriers to leaving?"

"Got it."

"The goal is not to make you a good intern. It's to make you a good doctor."

And a good person, I wanted to add but didn't.

An hour later, I excused myself from the noontime electrophysiology lecture, straightened my necktie, and set out for the primary care clinic.

"If you get to the Tuberculator, you've gone too far," one of the medical students whispered, referring to the spacious subway elevator where a few indigent men had recently taken up residence.

I skipped down four flights of stairs and headed out of the air-conditioned hospital and into the fetid, pulsing summer air, arriving at the Associates in Internal Medicine (AIM) clinic a few sweaty minutes later. During orientation, I'd learned that this rather unassuming clinic, staffed by physicians-in-training at Columbia, serves the northern Manhattan communities of Inwood and Washington Heights. The history of this community was an immigrants' tale—at the beginning of the twentieth century, an influx of Irish immigrants arrived; in the late 1930s, European Jews took refuge here. And when our new class of forty interns showed up, the area was, much like the lower rungs of minor-league baseball, overwhelmingly Dominican.

Orientation had concluded with the community's sobering health statistics: one in five adults in this neighborhood was obese. Half did no physical activity. Residents were nearly one-third more likely to be without a regular doctor than those in New York City overall, and one in ten went to the emergency room when they were sick, or simply needed health advice. "Welcome to Washington Heights," the head of our department had said. "You will be doing a great service for this community." It was clear that primary care would draw on a unique set of clinical and interpersonal skills, ones that I had most certainly not yet fully acquired.

A young receptionist in the AIM clinic inspected my ID, scanned a marker board for my name, and showed me to my office. "Here you are," she said, opening the door to one of seven generic offices. In the left corner of the room, a slab of butcher paper sat atop an examining table. Above it, a cerulean blue blood pressure cuff was mounted on a cheese-colored wall. To my right was a large wooden desk and computer. My first doctor's office.

"Just a reminder," the woman said, "when you're done seeing the patient you present the case to the PIC. Then bring the paperwork to me."

"PIC?" I asked. Medicine was quickly becoming a word salad of acronyms.

"Physician-in-charge. Just down the hall."

"Ah, the—"

"Yes." She winked. "The real doctor."

I had shadowed a primary care doctor for a month at Mass General and had the gist of how the system worked, but I knew it would be a mistake to assume the work in the clinic would be straightforward. If it was challenging for Baio, I didn't want to consider what my experience might be like. Fortunately, there was a real, board-certified primary care doctor, the PIC, just down the hall, in case I became confused or overwhelmed.

I logged in to the computer and found my patient panel. I was scheduled to see patients in thirty-minute increments from 1:00 P.M. until 4:30 P.M. Opening the medical record of my first patient, I felt a small thrill as I prepared to jot down notes about him, a fifty-three-year-old man who had been coming to the clinic for several years. I opened the last note from the previous primary care provider. But as I read, my eyes almost instantly went crossed. The note began:

Problem List

1. HTN
2. CKD

3. CAD
4. TIA
5. COPD
6. GERD
7. PVD
8. Migraines
9. ED
10. DM2
11. BPH
12. Active tobacco use
13. Depression
14. HLD
15. OSA on BiPAP
16. Afib on Coumadin
17. Glaucoma?
18. HCM: needs c-scope

What kind of patient had eighteen different problems to deal with? It seemed like I'd need a team of specialists in the room with me just to provide primary care. Sifting through the befuddling acronyms, I felt my stomach turn. I recognized some of the letter combinations, but every unknown acronym felt like a small knife in my side. Were they using a different set of abbreviations at Columbia? I suddenly missed the immediacy of surgery, of just fixing something right then and there, showing Axel, and moving on. I reread the note from the beginning and began Googling the various combinations of letters that weren't immediately recognizable.

My palms broke into a light sweat as I typed. What if this patient had other problems—problems that weren't on this list? Patients were more likely to focus on things they could feel, like a sore knee, than on things they couldn't, like diabetes or high blood pressure. How could I possibly address old issues and new ones in one short clinic visit? While the computer performed the search, my thoughts drifted back to Carl

Gladstone, as they had every time I found myself with a moment of free time. *Was he going to be okay?*

I had to say something.

After twenty distracted minutes I was only a third of the way through the patient's medical record, but sitting behind the large desk I did feel somewhat like a real doctor, at least more than I did in the cardiac care unit. Feeling a moment of modest inspiration, I hopped up from my swivel chair and decided to test out the blood pressure cuff. In medical school I'd always found the contraption cumbersome and knew from experience that fumbling with it would be a dead give-away that I was new in town. Once satisfied that I could hold the stethoscope in place with one hand while pumping up the cuff with the other, I returned to the medical record. After fifteen more minutes of referencing and cross-referencing, I had to shut my eyes.

Was it really possible to memorize and retain all of this knowledge? And more important—was it necessary? Or did real physicians retain a core of crucial information and simply look the rest up on the fly? Baio seemed like he'd seen it all before, drawing on experience to guide his decision making. As I dug deeper into the chart and all hope of diagnostic parsimony appeared lost, there was a knock at the door. I sprang up from my chair and opened the door.

"Dr. McCarthy," the receptionist said, "your one P.M. is here."

"Okay," I said. "Great."

"Do you want to see him?" she asked.

As I glanced at my notebook, I momentarily wondered whether any answer besides yes would be acceptable. In truth, I thought I'd need another hour before feeling prepared to see the patient.

"Well," I said, folding my arms, "I suppose I should—"

"It's one forty-seven P.M.," she said. "He was almost an hour late and your one-thirty P.M. just arrived."

"He seems kinda sick," I said. "Maybe we could do a shorter visit or—"

"I'll send him in," she said and closed the door.

A moment later, a stocky bearded man in a faded barn jacket entered the room and extended a callused hand.

"Sam," he said firmly.

"Matt. Mr. McC——Dr. McCarthy. Please have a seat."

I waved my hand across my desk like I'd just performed a magic trick. "You actually gave me some time to familiarize myself with your chart."

The fact that Sam was even upright and walking into my office under his own power came as a small surprise. After reading the long list of conditions in his chart, I was expecting a borderline invalid, but Sam looked rather well. He was husky, with shaggy gray hair that drooped into his eyes, and if Heather saw him on the street she might whisper to me that he looked like a sheepdog. "Terribly sorry I'm late," he said. "Didn't know you guys still used charts."

His smile revealed crowded, champagne-colored teeth. "It's mostly computerized," I conceded, "but yes, some records are still on paper."

In medical school they often filmed us interviewing an actor who was pretending to be a patient, to get a better sense of our bedside manner. I'd routinely been given the feedback that my somber demeanor was depressing to patients. I flashed a large smile and cracked my knuckles.

"There's a lot here," I said as I pointed at the monitor. "Seems like you've been through a lot. So . . . how are you?"

It had been drilled into my head to lead with an open-ended question.

"I'm good," he replied. "Real good. Feel great."

We sat in silence and I began counting in my head. I'd recently been reminded that most doctors interrupt their patients eighteen seconds into the interview. I nodded and opened my eyes wide, encouraging him to speak.

"You?" he asked flatly.

I finished counting to twenty and said, "Me?"

"Yeah, you good?"

"Yes."

I nodded and he nodded. There were many nods.

"So, let's get down to it," I said. "Now, I went through your chart and counted more than fifteen medical conditions. Since we're new to each other, I'd like to go through each one with you."

"Fifteen? That can't be right. I'm just here for a checkup."

"I agree it's a lot. It might be easiest for me to just go down the list. First on here is high blood pressure."

I was using an old improv technique to prolong conversation: avoid negatives; agree and add on. I glanced at the blood pressure cuff.

"Huh. Blood pressure is always normal. I wouldn't say I have high blood pressure."

"You take a medicine for it, yes?"

"Yes."

"Otherwise it would be high, no?"

He shrugged his shoulders. "I don't know. Maybe we should try."

"Try what?"

"Try not taking the medicine. Maybe my blood pressure wouldn't be high."

"No, it would."

So much for improv.

"Okay, next on here is kidney disease."

He shook his head. "No one has ever mentioned that I have kidney disease."

That seemed impossible. If the previous physician had put it in the note, why wouldn't he tell Sam about it? Or was there something about Sam I was missing—he wasn't responding to me in the way I had seen patients respond to primary care doctors at Harvard. Perhaps I needed to switch tactics—to change gears entirely—but how? In time I'd learn to ask wide-ranging questions—*is that growth on your face new? Is your diarrhea frothy?*—but for now, sitting in front of Sam, I was stumped.

A voice from outside the door announced, "Your two P.M. is here. One-thirty is still waiting."

My pulse quickened. "Okay, let's hustle through these conditions."

"Hustle away."

After twenty more minutes of stilted interrogation that produced little useful information, I stood up. Sam was clearly more confused now than when he'd arrived. "I'll be right back. Just need to discuss your case with someone. I'll be just—"

"Aren't you going to examine me?"

I looked down at the stethoscope that was resting comfortably on my desk. "Yes, of course."

The idea, undoubtedly, was that I would eventually find my way, stumbling upon a bedside manner through trial and error. But how long would that take? In orientation, the expectation of primary care clinic had been clearly laid out: residents would concoct a plan of action for each patient and the PIC would critique that plan, ensuring that the patient received quality care as we learned. I had supervision, but it was in another room, a room that at the moment seemed very far away. Every patient was trouble, the comatose ones who needed to be kept alive, the seeming healthy ones who might be dying, all of them my responsibility. Getting the adrenaline going was the only thing that momentarily relieved the pressure, but in the low-key setting of the clinic, my anxiety expanded to fill the room. And I suspected Sam could tell.

"Take a deep breath," I said, pressing my stethoscope against Sam's back. "And again." I took a few deep breaths, too, hoping it would calm my nerves.

As I searched in vain to find Sam's thyroid gland, which was supposed to feel like a bow tie, I missed Baio's silent hand gently pointing me in the right direction.

10

A few minutes later, as Sam waited, I walked down the hall to an office labeled PIC. Inside the room, a fifty-something man with a pageboy haircut was reading the latest issue of *The Journal of the American Medical Association.*

"Hello," I said softly, "I'm one of the new interns."

He put down the journal and looked up at me, beaming. "Welcome!" he said. "Please take a seat." The PIC, whose name was Moranis, was wearing khakis and a blue Ralph Lauren button-down with a red tie, the unofficial uniform of an academic physician.

"I want to apologize for running late. My first patient is a bit complicated."

Moranis shook his head. "Never begin any presentation with an apology. It's your first day in primary care," he said, quickly blinking his sea-green eyes, "and they're all complicated."

I took out my notebook. "Where should I begin?"

"You tell me. I'm just here for guidance."

I gazed down at the sun-faded notebook—a tempest of composition—and felt unsteady. "Well, I made a problem list."

"Good way to start. What's at the top of the list?" It was clear he'd been coaching young physicians for years, and I felt a bit more at ease. But that might've been just because I was no longer dealing face-to-face with a patient.

"Top of the list is high blood pressure," I said. "His blood pressure is a bit elevated today."

"Is he on a diuretic?"

I scanned the medication list looking for Lasix—the only diuretic I could think of. A day earlier, I'd mentioned on rounds that Lasix gets its name from its duration—"(la)sts (six) hours." Baio had one-upped me, detailing the way Lasix found its way into horseracing after it was noted to prevent horses from bleeding through the nostrils during races. Hence the term "piss like a racehorse."

"No Lasix," I said. "But he is on a bunch of other medications."

"Is he on hydrochlorothiazide? And do you know why I ask?"

"No. And no."

"Several years ago a large trial called ALLHAT showed that patients with high blood pressure should be started on a thiazide diuretic if single therapy is being initiated and another medication is not indicated."

"Gotcha." I quickly wrote down *ALLHAT.*

"However, you said this patient is complicated, so a different medication may be indicated. Perhaps Lisinopril if he has kidney . . ."

I tried to transcribe his thoughts but couldn't keep up.

". . . However, if he has heart disease a beta-blocker may be indicated."

How would I ever remember all of this? Did I have to go back and explain it to Sam? Maybe this was why the previous physician hadn't told Sam he had kidney disease—because it was just too complicated to explain.

As the waiting room continued to fill up, Moranis went through each of the issues on the problem list and explained the rationale behind each diagnosis and treatment. Despite the boyish haircut, he had the unmistakable patina of age and authority, and he spoke with a kind of joyfulness as he turned over each piece of information to examine the possibilities as they related to Sam. I tried to absorb it all but caught myself zoning out, watching his lips move while wondering if a lifetime spent memorizing journal articles and acronyms would turn me into someone like him. Someone who seemed to know more about my patient than I did without ever having examined him. Or would I become a creature so consumed by minutiae that I'd be incapable of interacting with patients on even the most basic level? Would it all just become a tangled skein of factoids?

"Let's go see your guy," he said finally, rising to his feet. "The best part."

When Moranis stood up, I realized that I could rest my chin on his head. This man whom I found so intellectually imposing was nearly a foot shorter than I was. As we walked back down the hall, I noticed that his eyes sparkled a bit the way Baio's did. I was with yet another doctor who felt squarely in his element. Would I really ever get to the point where any of this might seem pleasurable?

"This is my boss," I said to Sam as we reentered my office, "the physician-in-charge."

"Sam," he said, extending his right hand. "Your liege was just telling me all the things that are wrong with me."

Moranis turned his head toward me and frowned. "I understand you two covered a lot of ground."

"Dr. McCarthy mentioned that I have more than fifteen problems. Never thought of myself like that, but I guess it's good to be aware of it all."

"Let me offer an alternate hypothesis," Moranis said, holding up an index finger like his kid-shrinking namesake, as if about to introduce a tween-condensing laser beam. "You were told you had high blood pressure at a young age."

Sam wrinkled his brow, and Moranis nodded gently.

"Perhaps. That sounds right," he said.

"And I'll bet you were offered a medication for it."

"I don't remember, honestly."

"And you didn't take that medicine."

Sam flashed a mirthless grin. "You're right about that. I didn't take anything until I turned fifty. And then it apparently all went to shit."

"Your untreated high blood pressure led to kidney disease, which further exacerbated your hypertension. This, in turn led to heart disease." Moranis glanced at his belt and silenced his pager. "The heart disease," he continued, "led to liver disease, which in turn contributed to your erectile dysfunction. And the erectile dysfunction contributed to your insomnia."

"Great," Sam said, "so what's the answer? Treat the blood pressure and it'll all go away?"

Moranis held his finger up to his lips so he could listen to Sam's heart and lungs with his stethoscope.

"It's not that simple," I said, eager to contribute. "These are all chronic conditions that will likely need to be managed, not cured."

My pager went off, and Sam covered his eyes with his right hand. "You know it seems like I see a different doctor every time I'm here. Every few months I start from scratch with someone. Can you be my permanent doctor?"

We had made a small connection. "Of course I can be your permanent doctor. I'm here for the next—"

"No," Sam said, motioning toward Moranis, "him."

Moranis removed the stethoscope from his ears and moved toward the door. "We're a team here. You're in good hands. It was a pleasure to meet you."

"There's one other thing I didn't mention to your boss," Sam said meekly once we were alone. "I guess I was embarrassed. But I ran out of Viagra a few weeks ago and was wondering if I could get a refill."

The Viagra commercial popped in my head—an attractive baby boomer sailing on a lake—with the voice-over "Do not take Viagra if you take nitrates for chest pain."

"Do you take nitrates for chest pain?" I asked.

"You tell me, Doc."

I scanned his medication list. "No." I imagined Sam trying in vain to get an erection. "Of course, I can get you a refill."

We wrapped up our session a few minutes later. On my way to give paperwork to the receptionist, I stuck my head into Moranis's office.

"Thank you," I said, "for that. All of it."

"It's why I'm here."

"Well, thank you."

"Meant to ask," Moranis said, putting down his journal. "Did you notice that he'd been incarcerated?"

I was shocked. "Uh, can't say that I did. I suppose I got caught up in—"

"Quick tip. You can't just go through the most recent notes to understand your new patients." Moranis must've combed through the older notes while I was examining Sam. But there were dozens of notes in the chart. How did he know which ones to read?

I considered Sam, the adorable sheepdog. "Did you ask him why he was in jail? Did I miss that?"

A smile crept onto Moranis's face. "Why do you think?"

"I guess I'd be curious."

"Why?"

"I don't know—if he was a pedophile or serial killer or something?"

"Why?"

"You're asking me why it would matter if he's a sex offender? Or a wife beater?"

"Sure. Would that change anything about the way you treated him?"

The question sent my mind back to Boston three years before, to a seminar I once took at Harvard. One afternoon per week, a small group of students would get together to discuss prejudices in and out of medicine in a course called Emerging a Culturally Competent Physician. At the end of the seminar, we were asked to divulge one prejudice to the group.

"I think fat people are lazy, sometimes," a young woman said.

"When I hear a Southern accent, I kinda think the person might not be too bright," said another.

We continued in this manner until we reached Ben, an aspiring trauma surgeon like Axel, who was gently shaking his head.

"Frankly, I think we should all cut the bullshit," he said.

The professor raised an eyebrow. Ben possessed a swagger not seen elsewhere on campus; his was an intelligence we would never quite understand or possess. And he was one of Charlie McCabe's favorites.

"I think it's great that we're all sharing today," Ben continued. "I am friends with Matt," he said, pointing in my direction. "I like him and I look forward to hearing about his prejudices. And there's no doubt Matt here thinks fat people are lazy."

Heads spun toward me; I was mortified. I shook my head and mouthed "no."

"But I also have no doubt Matt would care for a fat person the same as anyone else."

I enthusiastically nodded.

"So who cares?" Ben said. "I'm more interested in the . . . the bad people in this world. What about a child molester? Should I operate? Should I try my damnedest to save the life of a monster?"

"Well," a petite future surgeon named Marjorie said, "I think we all bring certain values to the table that are inescapable. I know I won't treat every single person exactly the same."

"Oh?" Ben said.

"I . . ." She glanced down at her desk. "I couldn't treat a Muslim, for example."

Her Orthodox Judaism was no secret to the class.

Ben smiled. "Go on."

"But I know enough not to put myself in that position," Marjorie continued. "I would recuse myself."

"And what if you don't have that luxury?" Ben asked. "What if you're in a small hospital and you're the only surgeon?"

"I wouldn't let that happen."

"We're being trained to put people back together again," Ben said, scanning the members of the room. "We're not here to be a judge. Or to be a jury."

Marjorie shook her head. "I am just being honest."

"But perhaps," Ben said lightly, pointing an index finger at Marjorie, "perhaps an executioner."

"That's not fair, Ben. As I said, I was just being honest."

"I'm gonna go out on a limb," he continued, "and suggest you weren't this honest in your med school interviews." She did not answer. Ben turned to me. "Somehow, Matt, I bet it didn't come up."

I took a step toward Moranis and said tepidly, "Do you know why Sam was in prison?"

"I do."

"And?"

"It's in the chart."

"I might take a look."

"Feel free."

"I also wanted to mention that after you stepped out, he asked me to refill his Viagra. Didn't see any reason not to. I think he was a little embarrassed to bring it—"

"Sam was convicted of sexual assault eleven years ago."

I took a step back. What I knew about Sam after an hour in his file was almost nothing. But there was no way to discuss his personal life when I was still trying to wrap my head around the acronyms that spelled out his medical history. What if Sam was convicted of a crime, served his time, and was now married with a family? Or what if he was a monster?

"So," I said softly, "should I not refill the Viagra?"

Moranis smiled. "That's your call. He's your patient. I'm just here for guidance."

"Right. So . . ."

"So."

"How would you guide me?"

He stood up, put an arm on my shoulder, and said, "I would advise you to think about it and make the decision on your own."

I hung my head. This scenario must've come up before. What was the right answer? Was there a right answer? Why wasn't it all as simple as "Don't give the sex offender hard-on pills" or "Hey, that was a long time ago, of course it's probably fine"? And in any case, how could I be expected to make snap judgments on moral questions that might take days to sort through when I couldn't even manage to keep track of the patient's symphony of actual medical ailments, the stuff he truly needed me to be on top of?

I opened my mouth, but Moranis cut me off.

"The waiting room is filling up," he said. "You better get moving."

11

Several days had passed and I still hadn't mentioned Gladstone to anyone. And it was eating me up inside. Would there be repercussions? What would happen to him? Or to me? There were so few people I could talk to about this, so few people who would understand. Fortunately I lived with one of them.

"I fucked up," I said as Heather poured cereal into a bowl. "I really fucked up."

It was before dawn and we were both bleary-eyed. She wrinkled her brow and reached for a spoon as I continued talking, explaining the case of Carl Gladstone in painstaking detail. Reliving the moment was in no way cathartic; it only made me upset. As I had sufficiently laid out the case against my competence, I glanced at the clock. It was time to leave for work.

"The important thing," Heather said, "is that you told someone."

"Yeah, but that doesn't change what happened. The guy could've died. The guy *should've* died."

"But he didn't." She dropped her spoon and put her soft hand on mine. "You did what you were supposed to do. You didn't keep it to yourself."

I shook my head. It didn't matter. "This is killing me."

"Imagine how many people examined him and didn't even look at the pupils."

"But I did."

We ate our Cheerios in silence; my head pounded like I was hung-over, but I hadn't had a drink in days. Possibly weeks.

"You can't beat yourself up over this."

I knew she was right. I knew these things could happen. But I couldn't recall her making a mistake. I didn't remember her dealing with a grave error.

"Yeah," I said.

She looked into my eyes and smiled. "You're a good doctor, Matt. Remember that."

We slid our bowls into the sink, grabbed our white coats, and headed to work.

An hour later I was back in the unit, scampering from one room to the next, acquainting myself with the five new overnight admissions. The turnover was dizzying; it would take me hours to get up to speed. Denise Lundquist—the woman for whom the death of a sibling had triggered a heart attack—was now off the ventilator and would likely be transferred out of the unit before the weekend. One constant, however, was Benny. There he was, hour after hour, riding the stationary cycle or watching TV on his bed, as though he were someone whose small apartment just happened to be in the middle of a cardiac care unit. For a man with a diseased, failing heart, he had a remarkably good attitude, which made checking in on him a nice break from the rest of the unit's tense atmosphere. This morning he was watching an episode of *House* when I passed his room, which seemed a little bit to me like watching a disaster movie on an airplane.

"You good?" I asked, giving him the thumbs-up sign as I stuck my head in the door.

"I suppose."

"Excellent." I started to close the door and looked down at my scut list. There were thirteen more things to check off before rounds. I repeated his response to myself: *I suppose.* That didn't sound like Benny. I looked up and saw that he was wearing the same Giants T-shirt and hadn't shaved in several days. His beard was much whiter than I'd expected, and drops of sweat were gathering above his thin lip.

"You got a minute?" he asked.

"I have a minute. Less than a minute."

He muted the television. "Matt, I see a new group of interns in here every month. And when the moment strikes me, I like to offer feedback."

"Oh." In my limited experience, impromptu feedback was rarely welcome or constructive.

"Matt, just sitting here, waiting, I encounter all types. Good, bad . . ." His voice trailed off. "Mostly good."

"That's nice to hear."

"The good, the bad, but not the ugly." He chuckled to himself and fixed his eyes on mine. "Matt, you come across like you're always in a hurry."

"That's because I am." My spine unconsciously stiffened.

"Seems like talking to me or to just about anyone is another box to check for you." He lowered his head. "I'm just saying this because I know you're young."

"And impressionable," I whispered. I relaxed a little bit. This kind of criticism was hard for me to take. Not knowing stuff as a young, inexperienced doctor was one thing, but no one wants to hear that his patients think he doesn't care about them. Still, Benny's comment didn't feel like a dressing-down; his voice had an off-the-record feel that put me at ease. I sat down in the chair next to his bed and exhaled. "No, you're right," I said. "The truth is I feel completely overwhelmed."

"It kinda shows."

"Ha. Great. So much for never letting 'em see you sweat."

"But it doesn't have to."

I shook my head. "I suppose I should just get here even earlier."

"It's not about that. Not about that at all. Take a look at what you're doing. You're sitting down and we're having an actual conversation. Normally you just—"

"Plan an escape route the moment I enter the room."

"Yeah. And half the time you're looking at your papers or over your shoulder and not listening."

"But I am listening."

"Perception is reality, Matt."

Why was he sweating so much?

"What about you?" I asked. Was he sicker than I'd realized?

"Good days and bad days," he said. "Today's not so great."

I couldn't imagine being in his position, just waiting day after day. I'd be outraged. Unless his condition wasn't as stable as I'd supposed.

"You do look a bit warm," I offered. "Let's make sure you don't have a fever."

As I placed the back of my hand against his moist forehead, there was a knock at the door.

"Happy hour's over," Baio said. "Let's talk."

"Thanks for looking out for me," I said to Benny as I backed out of the room. "I'll get a nurse in here."

"Wasn't primary care clinic painful?" Baio asked as we walked to a pair of unoccupied computers. He was right, it was painful—but for a different reason; what I found overwhelming, he found boring. I studied Baio's face, wondering if he was ever going to bring up Gladstone. "Anyway, it's gonna be a busy day. Ridiculously busy."

I didn't want to think about it. I took a deep breath and reached for a bagel. With each day that went by without my being called to account for Gladstone, it was that much easier to just move on. I had been tearing myself up but had started to reach a kind of numbness about it. I just couldn't keep worrying or else I'd never get on track with the rest of my work, and probably completely destroy my stomach in the process. And as time went by, and no word came back from my superiors, it was easier to think that I might've blown up the whole incident in my mind. There was too much to lose in my bringing it up. In any case, Gladstone was undoubtedly in better hands now, wherever he was.

"You know," I said to Baio as my cointern Lalitha, a tall, attractive woman with a hint of a British accent and originally from Bangladesh, zipped past me, "I really marvel at these gals."

Lalitha was transporting Denise Lundquist to CAT scan while my other two pod mates, Ariel and Meghan, performed a paracentesis on one of the new admissions.

"Look at them," I went on. "Bright, energetic, enthusiastic, bouncing around the unit doing a hundred things at once." It hadn't been formally acknowledged that they were outperforming me, but I sensed they were, and constantly searched for signs.

Baio smiled. "Just remember everyone breaks." The smile disappeared. "Everyone."

"How so?"

"You can only shovel shit with a smile on your face for so long."

"Until what? Did you break?"

He swiveled around in his chair. "No comment. But speaking of shoveling shit, I need you to guaiac someone for me."

"Sure thing." Baio wanted me to insert my gloved finger into the rectum of a patient to assess for internal bleeding. I wondered if he needed to sound so pleased about it.

"Time to rectalize," he said. He patted me on the back. "You ever done one before?"

"Well—"

"I'll take that as yet another no. Honestly, did they teach you anything at Harvard? Anything?"

"I've done one before. But it wasn't on a patient."

Baio rubbed his hands together and grinned. "Oh, Dr. McCarthy, please do tell."

"Well, there's not too much to say. In med school a guy whose father had died of prostate cancer worked to help medical students learn rectal exams by being a kind of all-purpose guinea pig. Pretty much our whole class had a finger up his ass at some point. Nice guy."

"Whatever they paid him, it wasn't enough," said Baio. "But frankly, of the handful of practical things that they taught you at Harvard, I'm shocked that this was one of them." He waved his hand. "Anyway, I want to anticoagulate one of the new admissions. And before we can start a blood thinner, we have to make sure she's not bleeding internally. That's where you come in."

Just then a voice blared over the intercom: *ARREST STAT, FIVE GARDEN SOUTH! ARREST STAT, FIVE GARDEN SOUTH!*

In a flash Baio was gone. I leaned back in my chair and imagined him saying "ABC, ABC" as he sprinted down the corridor. He returned twenty minutes later, daintily holding his hands below his chest like he'd just received a manicure.

"Follow me," he said faintly.

He looked washed out, like something terrible had happened. Fortunately I saw no sign of feces on his scrubs. He led me to the back of the unit and into the residents' workroom—a cluttered space with half-eaten bologna sandwiches and potato chip wrappers strewn about two black leather couches. "Feel these," he said, keeping his eyes trained on his hands. "Go on, feel 'em."

I looked for a smile, a sign that he was joking, but there was nothing. I reached for his hands and rubbed his fingertips.

"This is weird, dude," I said, checking to see that no one was watching us. "What happened out there? And why am I rubbing your hands?"

"These, my friend, are healing hands."

He held them up and walked toward the floor-to-ceiling window overlooking the Hudson.

"Take a look at this." He motioned me to join him. "Over here." He pointed to small white marker board with a list of names, including his, running vertically down the left border. Across the top were four letters: ASDP.

"*A*," he said, slapping his finger against the board, "is for arrest. Number of arrests each one of us has responded to this month."

"You keep track?"

"Indeed. *S* is for survived. The number of people who survived those arrests."

"A scoreboard," I whispered to myself.

"*D* is for death."

"And *P*?" I asked, looking at the final, empty column. "Partial resuscitation? Paralysis?"

Baio laughed. "*P* is a category I made up just the other day. It's for pooping. The number of arrests called while the first responder was in mid-poop. Sadly, the number remains at zero."

I blinked. "Wait, what?"

"You'll notice, Dr. McCarthy," Baio continued, "that there are eleven slashes in both my *A* and *S* columns."

"I do. Eleven arrests, eleven survived."

"And that the column labeled 'deaths'—that column is conspicuously empty."

The other physicians on the list had a save rate just over 75 percent, a remarkable figure compared with national averages. But Baio was in uncharted territory.

"You've saved everyone."

I stood before him, awestruck.

"Not bad," I said, hoping to draw him out more.

"There's going to be a moment this year, many moments actually, when you'll ask yourself why you went into medicine," Baio said. "The year is going to knock the wind out of you."

"I believe it."

"I want you to remember this moment," he said, fighting back a smile. "Because it feels damn good to see a big goose egg up there under deaths."

"I will. I certainly will." Yet again I found it hard to believe that he had been in my position just one year earlier; what sort of process could transform me into him? I quickly estimated that I was learning between twenty and fifty new facts and one new procedure every day. Stretched out over an entire year, that was a lot of knowledge. But it still didn't seem like enough time. The learning curve would flatten and I'd certainly forget a few things. And I couldn't imagine that all of my instructors would be as gifted as the talented Dr. Baio.

"The lows in this job will be low," he said. "Very low. Unspeakably low. But the highs . . ."

"Yeah?"

"They're nice. The highs are quite nice."

12

He clapped his hands together like cymbals. "All right, enough celebrating. Back to work. Where were we?"

I followed him out of the room and back to the computers. "Before you left you said you wanted me to guaiac someone."

"Ah, yes. There are actually two treats in your future. Forgot to mention the M and M."

"M and M?"

"Morbidity and Mortality. It's a conference. Every so often we get the entire department together and go over a case where someone screwed up."

My mind instantly went to Gladstone. Surely his situation was tailor-made for unpacking at a conference that made case studies out of botch jobs. Could the case have made its way up the chain already? I knew about a small mistake or two made by one of my fellow interns, but nothing on the level of Gladstone, certainly nothing else worth exploring at length. In my mind, someone was holding a file folder marked "M and M" with a lone sheet of paper chronicling my idiocy. I was certain they were going to talk about me.

I might be able to drown my constant thoughts of Gladstone and my shame from Sothscott's phone call in the craziness of the CCU, but now I was forced to face the idea of a virtually public shaming in front of the entire department. What would the Badass think? Could any possible punishment or censure come out of it? My bowels shifted. I wondered if Baio could hear it.

"Jesus," I murmured.

"It's allegedly anonymous, but we can usually figure out who's responsible. Makes for high drama. Tempers flare, egos are crushed." Baio made a fist. "It's tragedy with a healthy mix of unintentional comedy. I'm always on the edge of my seat."

"Sounds awful." How could he be so fucking cavalier?

"Don't worry," he said. "I'll remind you about it later in the week. But back to the task at hand."

"Yes. Point me in the right direction of the rectal exam. I'm ready."

"Here's some guaiac juice," he said, handing me the developer that was to be applied to the stool. If blood were present, the brown fecal material would turn a brilliant blue.

"Thank you."

"No, thank you."

A nurse tapped Baio on the shoulder and whispered something in his ear. I applied a few drops of the developer to my finger to ensure there would be no mishaps with the actual stool sample. I sensed a moment to pick his brain.

"You said the lows this year would be really low." I rubbed the developer between my thumb and forefinger.

"Yep."

"But everyone says it gets better. Right? That it gets a bit better every year."

He scratched his chin. "They do say that, don't they? Well, I want you to know that they're wrong."

I wrinkled my brow. "Seriously?"

"All year people will reassure you that next year will be better. And the year after that. Trust me, it doesn't get better."

"Come on."

"Nope."

"I look forward to the day when I will actually feel like I know what I'm doing around here."

"That day ain't comin'. With more knowledge comes more responsibility."

"I suppose."

"You start taking your work home with you," he said, staring blankly at the computer screen. I wanted access to his inner world. Was he struggling in a way I didn't realize? Was he thinking of Carl Gladstone? Or was he just messing with me? I studied his face, but it offered no clues. Unlike so many doctors, Baio appeared unencumbered by anxiety or self-doubt. But what was beneath that highly competent exterior?

"Fine," I said, "I'm fine with that."

"Not fine. Okay, focus, Dr. McCarthy. I need you to rectalize room fourteen. Go with God, my friend."

The elevator door was closing several days later as Baio and I approached. He extended a hand and sprang it open, revealing a dozen white coats on their way to M and M—the Morbidity and Mortality conference. I thought about what I might say if Gladstone came up. I'd be contrite, certainly, but not defensive. I would acknowledge my mistake and accept the punishment and embarrassment that came with it. What else could I do?

"You can tell what type of doctor someone is by what they stick in a closing elevator door," Baio said as we squeezed inside.

"Oh yeah?"

"An internist sticks his hand. Surgeon sticks his head."

"And a social worker," said a woman in the back, "sticks her purse."

A six-three, rotund, bearded man in jeans and unlaced white tennis shoes flashed a grin and placed his hands on Baio's shoulders.

"Look who it is," he said, grinding his hands into the base of Baio's neck. "My first, my last—"

Baio wiggled out from underneath his grasp like a younger brother escaping a headlock. "What's up, Jake?" Baio threw a thumb in my direction. "This is my intern, Matt. Big Jake here was my first resident. Taught me everything I know—"

"When this guy showed up last year," Jake interrupted, placing a paw on my tricep, "he didn't know his ass from his elbow!"

It was impossible to imagine. "It's true," Baio said. "I was a mess."

"No," I said breezily. "No way."

"Oh yeah," Jake said, laughing to himself, "this guy was a total disaster!"

The rest of the elevator remained silent as I tried to imagine what his incompetence would look like. Baio racing around with fear in his eyes instead of assurance. Baio fumbling helplessly with primary care patients. Baio sitting on the other end of that miserable phone call from Sothscott. No mental image would stick.

The elevator reached the ground floor, and as we stepped out I realized Jake looked more like an offensive lineman than a physician. Perhaps he had been a football player; Columbia was full of ex-athletes. He slapped himself on the knee. "And now," he said to Baio, "you're telling an intern, another doctor, what to do? Amazing."

"Circle of life," Baio said flatly.

Jake turned to me. "Did he tell you about M and M?"

"A bit, yes." I didn't know what to make of this enormous oracle. "He said people get worked up. Something about egos getting crushed."

"And tears," Jake said, "don't forget about the tears."

"I'll keep my eyes peeled."

"Piece of advice," Jake said as he leaned in and nodded toward Baio. "Don't believe a word that guy says."

We took our seats in the auditorium, and I braced myself. Rapid-fire, shorthand conversations took place all around me, but a hush fell over the sea of doctors when a physician stepped onstage and tapped on the lectern's microphone.

"Welcome," she said, "to M and M."

I looked around the room, searching for signs of distress. I prayed they would not be discussing Carl Gladstone. It's been said that the first half of life is boredom and the second half is fear. If that's the case, I'd just reached middle age.

"Today, we're going to discuss a case with an unfortunate outcome. As always, I remind everyone that today's conference is confidential and—"

My pager went off: LUNDQUIST FAMILY WOULD LIKE TO DISCUSS DISCHARGE PLANNING. RETURN TO UNIT ASAP.

I took a deep breath, and another. I had to go but I couldn't get up. My ears were perked as the speaker ran through generalities pertaining to the M and M conference, tuned to any mention of the words "Gladstone" or "anisocoria." But the intro just dragged on. Baio looked over at me as I scanned the room, searching for other sets of eyeballs that might have drifted in my direction. The pager buzzed again. I had to go. I showed the message to Baio, shrugged, and excused myself, wondering if I was about to be lambasted in absentia.

13

I walked into Denise Lundquist's room and found her husband, Peter, seated next to her, gently stroking her hand with his own. Denise was asleep, and Peter, wearing a charcoal gray mock turtleneck and a pair of green jeans, had a legal pad in his lap. He was a young guy, probably in his early thirties, and he stood up quickly as I entered the room. I could tell he was flustered.

"Are you the attending?" he asked.

"No," I said, shaking his hand. "I'm the intern, Matt. I work with the attending."

I took a seat next to him, and he nodded, interlocking Denise's limp fingers with his. Something about his gentleness touched me. He was a solid, well-built man, but his voice was soft, almost a whisper, as if he were afraid he might wake his wife up.

"I have a bunch of questions," he said, touching the yellow pad. "Do you have a few minutes?"

"Of course, fire away."

I was conscious of my naturally somber demeanor and tried to lighten the mood with a large smile, but I wasn't entirely sure what I was smiling at. Denise was improving, but in rough shape. The hue of her skin still did not look human; it looked like it had been peeled from a mannequin. The situation didn't exactly call for confetti. Was there a proper physician's facial expression, I wondered, for a cautiously hopeful moment? Something that conveyed guarded optimism? I'd have to start watching Baio and the Badass for this.

Peter reached for his reading glasses on a small nightstand but, realizing he would have to let go of Denise to put them on, decided against using them. I motioned toward the bifocals, but he waved me away and cleared his throat.

"Today someone mentioned a possible heart transplant. Does she need a new heart?"

I stared at the young woman and squinted. Despite her terrible color, Denise was gradually improving, and on rounds we'd discussed transitioning her to a general cardiology floor in the coming days. Had Peter heard us talking about someone else?

"I'm not sure," I said. "I don't recall anyone mentioning a heart transplant for your wife. But I don't want to give you bad information."

"Understood." He checked off the first question and took a deep breath.

I leaned close to him and saw that he had written down thirteen questions. Instinctively I guessed that I'd be able to answer four, maybe five of them at best. I felt bound to disappoint Peter, or worse, leave him more confused, like I had Sam. As my jaw tightened for another round of teeth grinding, I suddenly became aware that I was moving almost imperceptibly away from Peter, toward the door. I had unconsciously sat back in my chair and could feel my legs tense, ready to rise; my body was beating an involuntary retreat. So this is what Benny meant, I thought. Looking at Peter looking at me, I could imagine what Benny saw: a doctor shutting down and going through the motions. A doctor who maybe didn't care enough. A doctor who was so afraid he might be wrong that he couldn't properly care for his patients. I caught myself and leaned forward, looking Peter in the eyes.

"I will obviously find out for you whether any heart procedure is being discussed," I said. "But I don't think there is."

Peter nodded. He stared down at the words he'd written on the legal pad but didn't speak. He simply stroked his wife's hand and watched her breathe. She made a faint gargle, and he parted his lips expectantly. I tilted my head to look at the questions, hoping I could read and answer them on my own. Squinting, I could just make out the next one.

Why did God let this happen?

Nope. I moved to the next one. Scanning down the sheet, I saw that he'd scribbled a heart and inside it written

Denise + Peter

I looked at this grief-stricken husband and then back at the sheet. In the bottom corner, he'd drawn a smaller, broken heart without names in it. Raising my eyes up from the drawing, I looked on as Peter wiped the bangs away from Denise's eyes.

And then, I burst into tears.

Not "eyes welled up" tears but genuine, blubbering, sloppy tears, heaving breaths, quivering shoulders. Perhaps it was the fear of what was being discussed that very moment at M and M, or perhaps it was being in the presence of such profound love and heartache. Maybe it was the lack of sleep. But the act of being there for Peter, of facing his pain and need, was simply too much. I had taken it all on myself and it flattened me like a pancake.

Peter led me by the shoulder to the corner of the room, gentle but urgent. "Matt," he said quickly, "is she . . . dying?"

I struggled to pull myself together. "No," I said through sobs. "Peter, she's doing amazing. Amazingly well."

He struggled to read my face. "Well then, what is it?"

My thoughts were with this grieving man, but they were also somewhere else. I ached to know what was being discussed at the Morbidity and Mortality conference. How many heads were shaking? Who was cursing my name?

"Denise is expected to make a full recovery." As the words exited my mouth, I wanted to snatch them back. I wasn't sure I was supposed to present such a rosy picture. On rounds, we agreed that Denise was improving, but she was still critically ill.

"Oh, thank God," he said, taking a step back. "Thank God."

"Yes."

My words belied my emotional state. Peter was very confused.

"You love your wife," I wanted to say.

I turned my blurry eyes in the direction of Denise and said, "It all got to me just now. I'm sorry."

He patted me on the shoulder. "We've all been through a lot."

I laughed the way one does through tears at a funeral. Here was another tip they'd omitted at medical school: when you can't comfort the patient, make the patient comfort you. Peter and I sat back down, and he once again took Denise's hand.

"Can we just sit?" he asked as he put the legal pad on her bed. "Just the three of us?"

"Yes, of course."

I was unaccustomed to such wild emotional swings; I wondered if I was developing a mood disorder. How did senior physicians build up enough emotional calluses to avoid bawling without becoming automatons?

"You know," Peter said, "it kills me to know I played a role in this." He touched the lobe of her ear with the back of his hand and frowned. "That I'm the one who told her about her brother. I keep replaying the scene in my mind, thinking I should've done it differently."

I wiped my eyes on my white coat as more tears trickled down my cheeks. I was a fucking mess. Everyone breaks, Baio had said. I just never guessed that I'd break so soon.

14

When I reconvened with Baio an hour later, I carefully watched his eyes for any sign that I had been the subject of M and M. But he never mentioned what was discussed at the conference and I never asked. I was too scared to. Its uneventful passing came to seem an absolution. We talked about our new patients, and that was it. Gradually, as the hours ticked by, Sothscott receded from the forefront of my consciousness.

"Listen," Baio said a few days later, "I got another person for you to rectalize. Room sixteen."

"Sure thing," I said and popped out of my chair. In those intervening days, I became increasingly proficient in a half dozen skills around the unit. Placing an IV was now a breeze, and I'd finally gotten the feel for dropping a nasogastric tube into a patient's stomach. "I can probably get it done before rounds." A modicum of proficiency in this task left me feeling exuberant. I pulled out the guaiac card and developer and shuffled toward room 16.

Baio's lips were pursed when I returned.

"What's up?" I asked. I caught the Badass out of the corner of my eye; rounds were about to start.

"That was fast," he scoffed.

I smiled. "No bleeding."

"You know you didn't even ask why you were doing that rectal."

"Check for bleeding," I replied. "And you asked me to." At this point, the job description seemed quite clear: carry out the will of the supervisor. Considering my relative ignorance, following his instructions to the letter was the safest course for my patients and for me.

"Right." We stood in silence, and he folded his arms. "And?"

I wasn't sure where this was going. "You ask me to do dozens of things."

"I do."

"And I try to do them as quickly and efficiently as possible."

Baio half-grimaced. "Enthusiasm is appreciated. But you're not thinking. You're doing."

"Yeah, lots of doing. Don't think. Do."

"Look, Matt, you're gonna spend the entire year being told what to do. A good intern will perform every task quickly and accurately."

"I'm certainly trying."

"But a great intern will pause and ask, 'Do these orders make sense?'"

"What do you mean?"

"Is it even necessary to guaiac someone before starting a blood thinner?" he asked.

I looked around the room. "Seems to be the standard practice in the unit."

"Are there any established guidelines that recommend it?" he asked disapprovingly.

It seemed like a reasonable thing to do, but I wasn't certain. I had learned a lot about advanced cardiac care in the unit, but I was no expert. "I'm not sure."

"Of course you're not. The point is that at some stage, you're going to be instructed to do something you shouldn't be doing."

What was he talking about? It was a frightening thought. What if all of my supervisors weren't as sharp as Baio? They were just one year ahead of me, and still in training. What if they struggled to perform procedures or were paralyzed by indecision? The implications were terrifying.

He patted me on the back and smiled. "I pray that you'll be able to identify those moments."

Rounds started a few minutes later. Ariel, the post-call intern, who'd been awake for twenty-seven hours, began by detailing the unusual condition that had brought the first of five new admissions to the unit. "Forty-one-year-old woman with nonischemic dilated cardiomyopathy and bipolar disorder on lithium was admitted to the CCU at four o'clock this morning."

Ariel had worked in consulting before applying to medical school, making the career switch in her mid-twenties. She was a star on rounds; her presentations were crisp, without a single wasted word. I imagined her in her previous life, standing before a boardroom in a pantsuit, telling executives that their company needed to cut out middle management and use less paper.

I sidled up to Lalitha's jet-black ponytail. "Hey," I whispered. "How's it going?" We'd been so busy paired off with our respective second-year physician-supervisors that there hadn't been much time for chitchat.

Lalitha stared ahead at Ariel and out of the side of her mouth whispered, "Barf." With her accent—was it Cockney?—the word sounded more like *boff,* which was slang for sex, and I bit my bottom lip so I wouldn't giggle. I, too, kept my eyes on Ariel—she was saying something about peaked T-waves found on the EKG—and wondered what Lalitha meant. What was "barf"? Was she feeling ill? Or was she referring to our jobs? Out of the corner of my eye the expression on her face was indecipherable. Was I barf? I was taking everything personally. Had I inadvertently done something to upset her? I glanced at Baio and thought about his "bumpy ride" comment.

I scribbled *What's barf?* in my notebook and placed it under her eyes.

"Everything," she whispered, her gaze still fixed on Ariel, who was trying in vain to place her tangle of red hair into a bun. "Has anyone considered," Lalitha said, now addressing the entire group, "that this is all lithium toxicity? It would tie everything together."

I certainly hadn't; it was a situation I'd only read about. Rarely did a day pass where I didn't find myself marveling at the brainpower around me. The hospital was filled with people with such different types of intelligence. Some appeared to have photographic memories, others were facile with logic and numbers. The interns and residents at Columbia were people who could do anything in life and they'd chosen medicine, working longer hours for lower pay, because it was important to them. It felt good to be surrounded by these people.

"Seems rather straightforward," Lalitha concluded.

Turning to me, she whispered, "Yesterday my resident had me draw blood on four people. Not cool." Doctors at other top hospitals weren't expected to carry out this time-consuming task, but at Columbia we were.

"Totally." I still couldn't reliably draw blood; Lalitha could do it in her sleep. She had gone to a medical school where students learned phlebotomy. I had not.

"And what do you think, Matt?" Dr. Badass bellowed. "Do you concur?"

I scratched my chin, unsure, but hoping to appear deep in thought. "I think," I said, "I think it would be a mistake to draw any conclusions before we finish hearing all of the details of this case."

Lalitha rolled her eyes.

"But," I said, "I'm tempted to concur."

Lalitha scribbled something on her scut list, then tilted it toward me and cracked a smile. I looked down to see the word *politician* with an arrow pointing at me. Perhaps she was right. Maybe I was just trying to give vague answers on rounds that couldn't later be used against me.

We stood in silence as Ariel presented the complex matrix of clinical information, repeatedly sweeping the frizzy red hair out of her eyes as the Badass pressed her to interpret the results of a transthoracic echocardiogram. Her sleepless composure was admirable; I knew I looked like shit after a night on call.

"All right, Dr. McCarthy," the Badass said at the conclusion of her presentation, "you have heard the entire case. What is your diagnosis?"

"Everything I've heard," I said as heads turned toward me, "points to lithium toxicity. Excess lithium led to kidney failure. Which in turn caused volume overload. Fluid overwhelmed the heart and lungs and she became—"

"Hypoxic," he said. "Very good. I agree. Next patient."

But I wasn't ready to move on. My mind had been churning Baio's advice—essentially to question everything—and as we prepared to move on to the next patient, I couldn't shake something that was nagging me about Ariel's case.

"But why?" I asked. Bodies froze mid-stride. I felt for a moment like a character in a network crime procedural. "It doesn't quite make sense," I added, looking from colleague to colleague. "Why was there too much lithium to begin with?"

"Overdose," said a pert, strawberry-blond medical student with a freckle on the tip of her nose.

Meghan, my third pod mate, shook her head. She had a kind, open face, with penetrating blue eyes. Like me, she had done laboratory research as a medical student, and at orientation we'd spoken briefly about becoming hematologists someday. She was from Dallas and had a well-concealed twang, which appeared only after she'd been awake for more than a day. "The patient has been on the same dose of lithium for twelve years," she said as she ran a hand through her butter-blond hair, "and has never had an issue."

"Suicide attempt," Diego, the brooding cardiology fellow, offered. "A call for help. Something like that."

"I spoke to her husband," Ariel said. "She's been in good spirits. Got a promotion at work. Looking forward to a vacation in Tuscany later this summer. I don't see her trying to kill herself."

"It's a good question," the Badass said. "And I agree, some aspects of the case elude explanation. Dr. McCarthy, I invite you to investigate it further after rounds. But in the interest of time we should move on."

Later I would realize his ruthless pragmatism was the only thing keeping rounds under four hours.

"Yes, sir. Will do," I said and scribbled *Lithium WTF!?!?*

After rounds, we gathered on the black leather couches and divvied up the day's remaining work. Diego and the Badass gave us this time to ourselves, to recover from rounds and to quickly eat lunch.

"Lalitha, I need you to draw a set of blood cultures on twelve," Baio said as he stared at the scut list he'd constructed over the past three hours. "And, Matt, transport the patient in four to CAT scan. Meghan, we need a central line on—"

"Why the CT?" I asked. I was on a roll.

He looked up from his sheet. "That was the plan we came up with on rounds. CT to rule out pulmonary embolus. Is that okay with you, Doctor?"

The other physicians and the medical student slowly turned toward me. I'd spent most of rounds surreptitiously reading about the diagnosis and treatment of pulmonary emboli in preparation for this moment. "The patient has all the classic symptoms of an embolus," I said timidly. "In critically ill patients, it's recommended to start treatment before the CT scan. Why are we waiting? Seems like we're wasting precious time."

Baio smiled; his style was disarming. "Good stuff, Dr. McCarthy. Anyone care to respond?"

No one spoke.

"Or is everyone here just mindlessly following directions?" he asked.

I glanced around the room; heads were down, fixated on impending scut. My face felt hot. I hadn't intended to implicate my cointerns as ill-informed automatons.

"When Matt heard 'pulmonary embolus,' he did the right thing,"

Baio said, clapping his hands. "He looked up the essentials of diagnosis and treatment. Well done. He looked in a textbook and attempted to make a clinical decision." It was strange to have our didactic sessions play out in front of others. I felt a creeping pride. "But he made a crucial mistake. He didn't then take into account the particulars of the patient."

My jaw clenched; I nearly bit my tongue. Baio was always one step ahead of me. *Don't run to the library when a patient is having a heart attack.*

"In this case," Baio went on, "if Matt had gone through the chart he'd've seen that this patient recently had a gastrointestinal bleed that almost killed her."

"Oh," I muttered.

He leaned over and patted me on the back. "Conventional therapy for a pulmonary embolus would likely kill this patient."

"Shit."

"But thank you for inquiring, Doctor."

Baio spun to the medical student. "Remember, medicine is not one-size-fits-all."

The student closed her eyes and said, "Of course."

15

A week later, Baio was in our lounge drawing a grid with the word *SHOCK* at the top when I decided to ask him a question that had been gnawing at me since we'd met. "How do you know so much shit?"

He kept writing, putting the finishing touches on his grid.

"It's like in one year," I went on, "you've—"

He spun toward me. "Okay, five minutes on the basics of shock."

"Photographic memory? Read a bunch of textbooks? What?"

"Flattery will get you nowhere, Dr. McCarthy. And sadly, medicine changes so fast most textbooks are irrelevant the day they're printed."

I thought of the textbook chapter I had slaved away at for months in medical school. "So what is it?" I persisted. Why was he being so opaque? I wanted to know what intern year had done to his psyche and how he'd apparently emerged unscathed.

Baio shrugged and stared out the window at a ship sailing south down the Hudson. "I guess you just see a lot intern year. And these little teaching things help. They help. You have to know your shit if you're going to teach."

"Definitely."

He slapped me on the shoulder. "Have to prepare yourself for all sorts of stupid questions."

"You know what they say," I said, "there are no stupid questions."

"Just stupid people," he concluded with a chuckle. "You know, you should be teaching."

"Me? Who?"

"Teach the medical student something. Anything. And never underestimate," Baio said, still fixated on the ship, "the power of humiliation. I still clam up when I see Jake. When I see some of the other docs. But they taught me so much it's absurd."

Was it enough to just show up every day? Were the daily experiences so dynamic and transformative that you had no choice but to learn medicine? I hoped so.

"I'll be right back," Baio said, leaping toward the door.

A moment later, Diego entered. He grunted in my direction and spent the next thirty seconds trying to decide if he wanted to eat an apple muffin or a cluster of grapes. I watched him from across the room. Diego commanded a lot of respect in our group. His not being Baio or the Badass put him in a position above me without quite being in charge of me, and though we didn't have a close relationship, I admired his intelligence. Diego's research had been published in some of the most prestigious cardiology journals in the world, but he preferred not to talk about it, telling me once that his work was "mostly boring bullshit."

Suddenly I heard myself speaking.

"Diego, do you, ah, do you remember Carl Gladstone? The professor from a few weeks ago?"

Diego selected the muffin and spun in my direction. "I do."

I held my breath, feeling like I'd just plunged deep underwater without an oxygen tank. Diego took a seat next to me.

"Do you know what happened to him?" I asked.

"Indeed, I do." His eyes grew wide, breaking through the squint. I waited for him to continue, but he didn't. I had considered every conceivable response to this question but still wasn't prepared for the answer.

"Is he okay?" I finally asked.

He put down the muffin and sighed. "Do you realize, Matt, that I was in the ER when Gladstone first arrived, or that I was the one who wheeled his ass to the cath lab or that I was the one who first noticed the pupils and called neurosurgery?"

I flinched and took in a short, quick breath, almost a gasp. "I had no idea."

Diego was right, I wasn't really sure how the CCU admission process worked. And I wasn't certain what Diego did with his day other than correct me on rounds. So what was Sothscott yelling about? Why that awful phone call?

"I got a call from one of the neurologists," I said meekly.

"Who was probably very fucking confused after reading your note. It was nonsense."

I tried to put the pieces of that first evening back together. Why hadn't Diego told me? Why hadn't I brought it up the next day?

"Why are you asking about him now?" Diego asked. "This went down weeks ago."

"I don't know." Why had it taken so long? Shame and insecurity.

Diego folded his arms and leaned back in his chair. "There's layer upon layer of supervision here, Matt. Even when you don't think anyone's watching . . ."

I folded my arms, mirroring him. "When did the neurosurgery consult happen?"

"While you were bullshitting with Benny."

Pressure rose in my head; my breathing became irregular as I thought of Gladstone's wife, Sasha. Things still weren't adding up. "What about my presentation on rounds? The Badass said to scan his head."

"I told him to cancel it. It had already been done." I recalled them whispering during rounds. "He went to the operating room right after your presentation—"

"Were you going to tell me any of this?"

Diego lowered his head. "Were you going to ask?"

I looked out of the window, thinking of Gladstone's pupils. What was the point in not telling me? It would've saved weeks of torment, weeks of anxiety. Was it just a test? Proving some kind of point? "Look, Matt," he said, "I'm not going to scream. I'm not going to throw things. But it's ridiculous that it took this long for you to ask about Gladstone."

I wanted to disappear. "I'm really sorry," I murmured. "I was embarrassed. I thought about Gladstone all the time."

Diego stared out onto the Hudson and took another bite of the muffin. "You have to ask yourself some tough questions in this job. But before you can do that you have to ask yourself a very basic one: Who are you looking out for?"

I slouched in my chair.

"Yourself?" he asked.

I extended my neck and shook my head. "Of course not. I—"

"Your reputation?"

"I just—"

"Or the patient?"

Searching for words, I thought about the promising medical student I had once been. I recalled the look on Charlie McCabe's face when I first sutured up the banana peel in his office and the disappointment, months later, when I told him I did not want to be a surgeon. And as I sat there, head in hands, I realized I had forgotten to send flowers to McCabe's funeral service, which had taken place earlier in the week.

As I sat there trying to process it all, Baio reentered the room.

Diego shook his head and stood up. "You really think we're gonna leave all the decisions to you two bozos?"

PART II

16

In medical school, after I'd broken the news to Charlie McCabe that I'd chosen internal medicine over surgery, he'd grimaced and said, "Let me introduce you to someone." I followed him across the Mass General lobby to another set of offices where a man named Jim O'Connell was embracing a middle-aged woman in pink tights, a pink sweater, and bright red lipstick that had been haphazardly applied far beyond her lips. O'Connell was about the same age as Charlie McCabe and looked like a dad on a network television show: neatly parted gray hair, kind eyes, cardigan sweater, and a broad, welcoming smile. He immediately put me at ease.

"Jim!" McCabe exclaimed as we caught sight of him. McCabe turned to me and threw a thumb at Jim. "Someone should write a book about this guy." Jim O'Connell waved McCabe's suggestion away and extended a hand.

Both men had done their residencies at Massachusetts General Hospital, and like it had with McCabe, life had thrown Jim a curveball when he finished his training. He had planned to begin an oncology fellowship at the Memorial Sloan-Kettering Cancer Center in Manhattan, but at the conclusion of his three-year internal medicine residency, Jim had been asked by an MGH administrator if he'd consider spending a year assisting with a new program bringing health care to the homeless. He agreed, and his one-year stint with the homeless turned into twenty-five. And in the process, he cofounded Boston's

Health Care for the Homeless Program and revolutionized the way health care was delivered to the indigent.

"Until next week, Jimmy," the patient said as she leaned in to hug him.

"Wouldn't miss it, Sheryl."

After the woman in pink stepped aside, McCabe asked Jim to explain his work to me. O'Connell summarized his career in the way one learns to do when soliciting donors is a way of life: after receiving a master's degree in theology from Cambridge, O'Connell came to a crossroads; he joked that his liberal arts education had left him "uniquely prepared for bartending and driving cabs." After bouncing around the country—teaching high school in Hawaii, waiting tables in Rhode Island, baking bread and reading in a barn in Vermont—he did the improbable and went to medical school. He arrived at Harvard Med at age thirty, around the time that Charles McCabe developed that first tingling sensation in his hands.

"Come out in the van with me," Jim said as I scanned his spartan office and he prepared to see his next patient. "Come out tonight and meet our patients."

It wasn't clear why he was making the offer, and I wasn't sure, as a medical student, what I could bring to his program. Perhaps he had a deal with McCabe—maybe guys who turned their backs on surgery had to pay penance by riding in the van with Jim. I turned to McCabe, who was smiling. "Do it."

Later that evening, I met Jim at one of Boston's well-known homeless shelters, the Pine Street Inn, wearing a crisp white button-down shirt, khakis, and a new Calvin Klein tie. Taking a seat in the corner, I looked on as Jim, dressed like Jerry Seinfeld in jeans, white sneakers, and a navy blue polo shirt, tended to a long line of men and women who were there to get their routine checkups. His unique skill, I soon discovered, was that he never cut anyone off. He let his patients ramble on about anything they wanted, mostly issues wholly unrelated to their health, while he poked and prodded, quickly and quietly looking into ears, noses, throats, and any other orifices in need of inspection. He was able to time the cadence of a story, applying his stethoscope when someone paused to catch his or her breath and removing it when the story resumed.

I wanted to take notes but there was nothing to write; he simply knew how to interact with each and every patient. And he was especially adept at interacting with people who clearly had mental illness. He knew the names of distant family members and the details of obscure conspiracy theories. His method was remarkable—there was something almost religious to it—like he was the priest and his patients were the confessors.

Hours later, after the last patient had been seen, Jim went behind the counter of the soup kitchen and loaded up two dozen Styrofoam containers with chicken noodle soup. From there, I tagged along as he hopped in a van and began seeking out Boston's homeless who, in Jim's words, were "temporarily off the grid."

Our driver, a Haitian man named Pierre, followed his normal route, stopping at ATM branches, abandoned subway stops, and indeterminate New England wastelands searching for people who might appreciate a warm meal, a pair of socks, or their blood pressure medication. We were seeking out the people I actively avoided in everyday life, the ones wearing rags who hadn't bathed in months. I couldn't believe there was a man—a Harvard Medical School faculty member, no less—who was on a first-name basis with the scores of otherwise nameless people we encountered. And without fail, they were glad to see him.

"Tell them something about yourself," Jim advised that first night as we walked with flashlights, searching for a man known to sleep near a riverbank. "Tell 'em anything. Just be yourself and be honest." Jim cut a solitary figure as he forged ahead to where water met land, waving his flashlight back and forth like a tiny lighthouse. He spotted a pile of blankets next to the Charles River and motioned me over. There was a shine on the water from distant construction lights, and I could feel my heart thumping with every anxious exhalation. Lifting his index finger to his lips, Jim whispered "All yours" and disappeared in search of others.

"Sir?" I said, staring at the pile of blankets that was gently oscillating like an accordion. "Hello? Hello there? Anybody?" I looked out over the river and frowned. "My name is Matt," I said, rubbing my hands together. "Just here to check in." I inched closer and placed my right hand on the pile of blankets. "I'm working with Jim O'Connell and Health Care for the, uh, do you know Jim?"

At that point in medical school, I was several months removed from the banana peel; there was no chance that Axel ever had to seek out patients like this. I began grinding my teeth as McCabe's voice trickled into my head: *Ask yourself a deceptively simple question: Can I imagine myself being happy as anything other than a surgeon?* Like a sine wave, the blankets bounced up and down as I considered my words. "Hello? Anyone?"

I was preparing to turn around when a voice emerged. Soon a pair of eyeballs was staring back at me.

"Hey," I said, "I'm Matt."

"You work with Jim? Is he here?"

I leaned in, trying to make out a face. "He is. Would you like me to get him?"

"Who are you?"

"I work with Jim," I said tentatively. "I'm a student. I brought socks and soup."

"Can I . . . can I talk to Jim?"

"Yes, I'll get him."

"Can he take a look at this?" The man emerged from under the blankets and pointed to an open sore on his left shin. The skin was dark and mottled, with pus weeping from the borders. The stench was overpowering and unforgettable; I fought the urge to turn my head away. "Let me get Jim," I said softly.

As I headed back to the van, I thought of the material I'd been stuffing in my brain during medical school and compared it with what was floating through Jim's head. He held in his mind an intricate map of the city's homeless, a human atlas that few, if any, possessed. Jim O'Connell was undoubtedly the only physician who could tell you why one overpass was preferable to another for a good night's sleep or why Copley Square was better than Faneuil Hall for panhandling.

And like Axel, Jim was happy to dispense wisdom. "The key," he said later that night as we walked with flashlights under a condemned bridge, "is to build a relationship. It's easy to condescend. Resist that urge." And after a challenging interaction, "The problem is us, not them." Between stops, Jim and I talked about Whitey Bulger, Boston's enigmatic criminal, and baseball. "Dennis Eckersley," Jim said, referring to the former Red Sox pitcher, "his brother was homeless. Who knew?"

I found myself coming back to my apartment in Brookline raving about the experiences. I wanted to be like Jim. I wanted to *be* Jim: an unconventional, understated, brilliant doctor who played by his own set of rules, engaging patients in ways I'd never seen or considered. His method tapped powerfully into my own self-image as an outsider—the pre-med who was a ballplayer, the Ivy Leaguer in the minor leagues. In medicine, too, I knew I wanted to be something different but I wasn't sure what that something was until I met Jim.

More than a few times, my roommates were subjected to my theory that Jim O'Connell was doing for Boston's poor what Paul Farmer, the subject of Tracy Kidder's book *Mountains Beyond Mountains* was doing for Haiti. "Do you know what he's building?" I'd ask Heather, referring to the centerpiece of O'Connell's oeuvre, a massive medical complex that included a 104-bed inpatient clinic and dental clinic designed for the homeless. "Do you realize," I'd say, time and again, "just how incredible that is?" My friends quickly tired of hearing about it, but I never tired of telling them.

One morning, I found myself in the corner of Jim O'Connell's small office at Mass General, looking on as he examined the middle-aged woman with smeared lipstick, the one he'd been speaking with when McCabe introduced us. This time Sheryl was wearing dirty gray sweatpants and a blue Tasmanian Devil sweatshirt. Neon lipstick was smudged across her lips and cheeks.

After removing his stethoscope from her chest, O'Connell sat down in a black plastic chair a few inches from Sheryl and took one of her hands in his. "Everything looks good," he said. "Very good. Things are trending in the right direction."

She looked over at me and in a stage whisper said, "I was hoping for great."

"Everything looks great," Jim added warmly. "Blood tests, urine test, heart and lungs. I couldn't be happier."

I had seen Sheryl at the Pine Street Inn several times and learned from Jim that she'd been living on the streets of Boston for nearly a decade. Sheryl tended to ramble about her ex-husband and occasionally burst into fits of laughter for no apparent reason. She once shouted at me about the television show *Designing Women*.

Jim gently pulled Sheryl's hand in his direction to regain her attention. "You know what I'm going to bring up next," he said. "And just because you say no doesn't mean I'm ever going to stop asking."

She leaned toward him and their knees almost touched. "Lay it on me, Jimmy."

He took a deep breath. "I would like you to speak with one of our mental health professionals." Sheryl pulled back slightly but left her hand resting in his. "This is not a judgment against you," he said. "I just think you'd benefit from talking to someone. Someone with more expertise than me." She closed her eyes as he continued to speak. "We've been talking about this a long time and I think it would really help. And the clinic actually has an opening today. You could be seen this afternoon."

I stared at Sheryl, wondering what was going through her head, as my eyes fixated on the lipstick. Why not talk to someone? What's the harm? I straightened my freshly starched white coat and folded my arms.

"I understand why you don't want to go," Jim said, edging closer to her. "Really. But this is important, and I'm not going to stop bringing it up."

She shook her head. "I'm not crazy."

"I know that. I know you're not crazy. But I still think this could help."

Sheryl looked down at the floor, and my eyes drifted in the direction of her gaze. What was she thinking? *Was* she crazy? In our brief interactions, it had kinda seemed like it.

"It's important," Jim added. "Really important."

Sheryl looked over at me, and I gave a gentle nod.

"Please consider it," he said.

She gave him an exaggerated smile and softly said, "Fine."

My eyebrows raised, and so did Jim's.

"I'll do it, Jimmy. Whatever you want."

"You will?" he asked.

"I will." Sheryl looked at me, grinning. "He has been a pain in my ass about this for years. Years! Never shuts up about it. *Go see someone. Go talk to someone.* Well, I'm talking to you, Jim! I'll talk all you want."

I wanted to respond but wasn't sure what to say. "Is that right?" I muttered.

"I'll make the referral now," Jim said, flashing a flicker of a smile. "Right now."

A moment later the appointment was over. Sheryl grabbed her belongings, gave Jim a hug, and said, "To be continued," as she sauntered out of his office toward the mental health clinic. When the door closed, I noticed that O'Connell was staring at a blank sheet of paper on his desk.

"Interesting lady," I said, approaching him. "Really interesting." I took a seat where Sheryl had been. "Lot going on there."

Jim sighed and looked at me. "That woman has had her life ruined because of mental illness," he said. "Her marriage, her job, every inter-personal relationship. All destroyed." His eyes became moist and his voice soft. "I have been trying for six years to get her to see a psychia-trist and she has always refused. Every single office visit for six years. Always said no."

I studied his face, trying to think of something significant to say. But I could only offer a single sound. "Huh."

"She has never given herself a chance." Jim pounded his right hand on his thigh and smiled. "Until today."

"Incredible." His eyes bounced from left to right, and I tried to follow them. I could hear voices just outside of the office discussing a new coffeemaker. "Why today?" I took out a pen and a small notebook from the front pocket of my white coat and started to jot down the details of the exchange. "Wonder what changed," I said.

I waited for Jim to say something about persistence or tact, but he didn't say anything. He just stared at the blank sheet of paper. As we sat in silence, I tried to imagine what the last six years of encounters with Sheryl had been like. Had she yelled at him? Politely declined his suggestions? Did he ever get frustrated or upset with her?

"Matt," he finally said, putting a warm hand on my shoulder, "sometimes things that on the surface can seem like small victories, very small victories . . ."

His voice trailed off, but I wanted him to continue. I put down my pen. "Yes?"

He stood up and shook his head. "Sometimes those things can ac-tually be tremendous victories."

I was so taken with Jim and his philosophy that I convinced Harvard Med to give me course credit for schlepping around with him. Instead of making me learn how to efficiently manage a complex primary care visit with a guy like Sam, the school gave me primary care credit for assisting Health Care for the Homeless one night each week. That's part of the reason I felt so overwhelmed when I started working in Columbia's primary care office; I had watched Jim provide primary care out on the streets, but I hadn't done much of it myself.

Sure, I dispensed clean socks and foot ointment and listened when people wanted to chat, but Jim was the one examining and treating people. He was the one making tough decisions, convincing a reluctant recluse to go to an emergency room or providing reassurance. But it was during those late-night rides that I discovered how important it is to connect with patients. He was the reason, I realized later, that I first went to Benny's room when Baio asked me to introduce myself to the patients in the CCU. I didn't gravitate to the most medically complex patients, I went to the guy on the stationary bike—the guy I could talk to and potentially connect with.

From Jim I learned that through medicine it is possible to reach the unreachable—even the ones who most of us forget about or actively try to ignore. This is the power and beauty of our profession. He spent his evenings with Boston's homeless so they would trust him, so they would come to his clinic when illness struck. And this, I discovered, was no small task for people who lived under bridges or in large boxes near abandoned warehouses—people who were embarrassed by the sores on their legs or the smell of their skin. To walk into a hospital's lobby in shambles and sit in a waiting room was not something most would even consider. But they did it for Jim.

And I wanted them to do it for me.

17

"Let's start with the basics," said a woman holding a marker outside of a patient's room. I had completed my month in the cardiac care unit, parted ways with Baio, and moved on to the infectious diseases service. My new assignment—tending to patients with HIV, tuberculosis, or viral hepatitis—was widely considered the most fascinating and emotionally taxing monthlong rotation of intern year, which was hard to imagine given what I'd just gone through. The majority of the patients checked in to the infectious diseases wing of the hospital, we were told, were intravenous drug users or had mental illness. They were the unreachable patients who might yell at you or spit at you, the ones with nothing to lose who would exploit any sign of weakness—emotional, professional, or otherwise.

"If a patient shows up in our emergency room and says they have HIV, what six pieces of information must you obtain without fail?" Dr. Chanel, a junior faculty member in the Division of Infectious Diseases, asked of our small group of residents and medical students. She was in her late thirties and had a gently graying side ponytail. Muffled whispers passed around the half circle. We had just emerged from the room of a young woman who had reluctantly come to our emergency room because of a persistent sore throat; Ariel had been the one to inform her that her symptoms were actually due to acute HIV infection while we all looked on anxiously. As tears streamed down the patient's face, I had been sent out in search of Kleenex. After a few minutes of fruitless searching, I had returned with a handful of paper towels and toilet paper, which the woman had waved away. Then we'd all shuffled out.

Our group now had a brief moment—a thirty-second huddle—to try to learn something from this encounter before we were sucked back in to the maelstrom of buzzing pages and relentless orders. "One," Dr. Chanel continued, "what year did they contract HIV? Is this someone who has had it for twenty-five years and been through numerous treatment regimens, or is this someone like our last patient, who contracted it a week ago and is struggling to cope with the diagnosis?"

I wondered if this moment would have been better spent counseling the woman who had just had her world upended.

"Two," Chanel said, as we took notes, "what is the CD4 count. This is the subset of white blood cells that HIV destroys. Three: viral load. This is the quantity of replicating copies of HIV in the blood. The goal, not surprisingly, is for the viral load to be undetectable. Four: risk factors. How did the patient get HIV?"

I half-raised my hand, and Dr. Chanel nodded at me. "Why does it matter *how* the person contracted HIV?" I asked. "Seems like they've either got it or they don't. Not really our business how they got it."

She scanned the group. "Can anyone answer Dr. McCarthy's question?"

Meghan cleared her throat, perhaps in an attempt to suppress her twang. "Well," she said, "patients who get it from IV drug use are more likely to have hepatitis C or endocarditis. Patients who get it through receptive anal intercourse should be screened for anal cancer."

Chanel smiled. I wondered if it was the first time that a sentence ending with the words *anal cancer* made someone do that. "That's exactly right."

I quickly jotted this information down, pausing once to consider how poised Ariel had remained while relaying the devastating diagnosis. I couldn't have done it as easily as she had. I wondered if her time in consulting had prepared her for delivering bad news. Possibly she was used to walking into a room, ruining someone's life, and walking out.

"Good. Point five," Chanel went on, "what medications are they on? Does their HIV regimen make sense? And six. What opportunistic infections have they had? HIV patients get bizarre infections. That's actually how the virus was discovered. Otherwise healthy gay men in the early nineteen eighties were developing—"

ARREST STAT, SIX GARDEN SOUTH! the intercom blared, and my knees buckled. *ARREST STAT, SIX GARDEN SOUTH!*

I was the only one in our group who visibly flinched. Recently I had resigned myself to the fact that the screeching, electrifying announcement was something I'd never get used to. Two members of the team sprinted away, and I thought of Baio, hustling to revive yet another person. It was strange being separated from him. I wondered where he was and whom he was teaching. The man who'd taught me so much over such a short period of time was now just a guy I passed in the lobby or caught wolfing down a piece of pizza at grand rounds.

"Perhaps we should stop there," Dr. Chanel said, readjusting her side pony. "Let's reconvene in twenty minutes."

A few minutes later, the second-year resident I'd been assigned to work with in this portion of my rotation, Ashley—my new Baio—returned from the arrest. She had impossibly high cheekbones and spoke in clipped, overcaffeinated sentences with one thought emerging in the midst of another. In retrospect, she gave the impression of Jennifer Lawrence on speed, perhaps with more sensible shoes.

Ashley had greeted me that morning by saying, "Don't do anything without running it by me first. Are we clear?" Before I could respond, she'd launched into the array of tasks that needed to be completed before rounds—rattling off assignments like wheeling a patient to dialysis and transporting a vial of blood to the chemistry laboratory—faster than I could write, and then withdrew the work delegated to me just as quickly, explaining that it was quicker if she just did everything herself. This was becoming a regular routine, and it made me feel expendable and potentially dangerous. It was clear she considered me a liability, someone who still couldn't enter computer orders related to HIV care or write notes as proficiently as she could. Our brief exchanges were reminiscent of a naughty child and a frustrated babysitter. Her friends called her Ash, but she'd instructed me to call her Ashley. The intentional distance she put between us made me anxious. Even though we were hardly a personality match, I wanted to click with her. I wanted to click with everyone.

"Where were you?" Ashley asked, running her hands through olive oil hair. "You're supposed to come to these arrests."

I looked up from my scut. "I didn't realize."

She flashed a stiletto stare. "Realize."

"I didn't see any of the other interns going so I—"

"I don't need an explanation. Woman's dead. Dead on arrival." Ashley shook her head. Baio must not have been there, I thought.

"We're reconvening with the attending in about ten minutes," I said.

"Good. Here's the deal. Very simple," she said quickly. "I understand your physical exam skills are quite good, but you, ah, need some work in other areas."

"Right." I wondered if the Gladstone episode had reached Ashley.

"So let's play to your strengths. You're the eyes and I'm the brain."

"Got it."

"Examine the patients, tell me how they're doing, and I make the plan."

I scribbled down *Me eyes/Ashley brain.*

"And then, Matt, you carry out that plan. Make sure shit gets done."

I no longer trusted myself to remember anything unless it was written down. There were literally hundreds of small tasks and new factoids that popped into my brain over the course of the day, and I found it impossible to keep track of them all without committing them to paper. And prioritizing it all required yet another set of skills. "Yes, ma'am," I said awkwardly. My daily scut list looked like a madman's diary, every inch covered in scrawl. I often thought of Axel, imploring me not to write on my hands.

"And if I can give you one piece of advice, it's this: be efficient."

"I'll do my best."

"But efficiency necessitates competency," she said. "There's too much to know. Information is generated so quickly. And at your stage you're still trying to learn the basics." Again, Ashley was right. Scores of scientific journals were constantly churning out new and at times contradictory medical information. We would never have time to read it all and were in need of a competent curator. In many ways, Baio had filled that role for me in the CCU. But I needed to do it myself now; Ashley didn't seem like the type who would spoon-feed me information.

A young man wearing just underwear walked by us, demanding to be read his Miranda rights. "To that end," I said, trying to ignore him, "I've actually started using UpToDate," referring to a website that summarizes expert medical opinion.

"Wonderful," she said. "It should be your bible."

"It's incredible."

"Just don't reference it on rounds—attendings think it's lazy."

Two nurses escorted the hallucinating man back to his room.

"Use it for everything but anatomy," Ashley said. "Netter for anatomy."

Netter referred to Frank Netter, the physician-artist whose medical illustrations are the standard for human anatomy. Ashley tapped her pen to her cheek and fought back a smile. "Being from Harvard, your anatomy skills must be, ahem, disastrous." She was referring to the worst-kept secret among top medical schools: a paucity of corpses meant Harvard students had to choose to dissect either an upper or a lower extremity but not both. I'd been a leg man.

"Guilty." I smiled. "I've actually been trying to read at home when I can."

"Don't," she commanded. "Reset your brain at home."

"Okay."

"Bust it here. But when you're home, you're home."

I thought of the mindless hours I'd logged at home since starting internship watching reality television and reading tabloids in the name of mental health. Our generation of physicians was undoubtedly different—it was hard to imagine the Badass doing something similar. Did he take a look at Baio and think *Happy Days*? Or *Joanie Loves Chachi*? Doubtful. Maybe he played golf or flew single-engine planes.

Ashley looked at her pager as she took a large gulp from her latte.

"You know," I said, feeling momentarily unguarded, "I continue to feel overwhelmed. Trying to wrap my head around everything and learn how to do procedures." I wasn't entirely sure why I was opening up to her, but chronic sleep deprivation led most of us to behave in unusual ways. I found myself more willing to confide in my colleagues; others burst into tears when the cafeteria was out of ketchup.

She frowned. "That's not something you should go around advertising."

"Just being honest."

"No one wants to hear that you're struggling. I certainly don't."

I flinched. "True."

"Be confident. You know more than you think. But enough with the teeth grinding." She held up an EKG. "Anyway, would you rather have a doctor who's right or who's certain?"

A moment later, a medical student named Carleton joined us. He was from Princeton. Or an Abercrombie & Fitch ad. Possibly both.

"Just spoke to Ms. Sarancha for an hour!" he said with a mix of enthusiasm and frustration. Medical students were first against the wall when a demented patient requested to chat with a doctor. At Mass General, an intern once sent me in to talk with a patient but neglected to mention that the man was capable of saying only one word: "Why?" After exhausting my meager explanatory skills, I picked up the patient's chart and realized he wasn't overly inquisitive; rather, he'd suffered a massive stroke that impaired the part of the brain responsible for producing language. As pranks went it was relatively harmless and ultimately built camaraderie between the intern and me. It was the kind of thing Baio would do.

"Thank you for doing that," I said to Carleton. "Morning's going to be busy, but let's spend a few minutes this afternoon talking about shock."

Ashley shot an unsparing look. "Why are you discussing shock?"

It was one of the few topics I had mastered, that was why. And because Baio told me I should teach. "Fundamental topic to discuss," I offered.

"To cover in the ICU," she said, "but not here. We should focus on learning all we can about HIV." In that case, I thought, Carleton was out of luck. I knew little about the virus, certainly not enough to teach. "That's how things stick with you," she said. "See the condition, read about it, and associate the patient's face with the condition."

"I just think it's—"

"This isn't a dialogue," she said, her distaste palpable. "That's the way to do it."

Ashley's approach was reminiscent of a drill sergeant. Even on our most hellacious days, it had never felt like Baio was crowbarring a teaching session into our dialogue; it just flowed naturally as we hopped from one patient to the next. But though their styles may have differed—Ashley seemed to talk down to me while Baio propped me up—both wanted to impart vivid images that I would never forget. Teaching points and patient scenarios that would stick in my brain for decades.

"Okay, Carleton," I said as Ashley picked up her phone, "if things calm down this afternoon we can talk a bit about HIV."

ARREST STAT, EIGHT HUDSON NORTH! ARREST STAT, EIGHT HUDSON NORTH!

Ashley and I shot out of our chairs and sprinted toward the stairs.

ABC, ABC

In the hallway, I darted past a bewildered Peter Lundquist, nearly colliding with the Tupperware container in his hand. Peter brought in cookies and cakes for the CCU staff day after day, even after Denise had been transferred out of the unit. They had been a delightful change from the pungent Filipino ginger desserts we were accustomed to.

When I reached the arrest, two dozen physicians and nurses were already at the bedside.

"Too many people," one of the nurses said. "People out now."

Intern orientation had introduced me to the concept that more physicians equals more chaos. I backed away from the lifeless body. A few steps past the door, someone grabbed my arm.

"Where do you think you're going?"

It was Baio.

"Too many people," I said, throwing a thumb toward the crowd.

He shook his head. "You never leave an arrest. Never." He escorted me toward the room. "If someone tells you to leave, you move behind a curtain. If someone pushes you back, stand in the doorway. You need to see as many of these as you can. Let's go."

We stood in the doorway, watching the madness unfold. "Michael Jordan said the game would slow down for him," Baio whispered, "when he was in the zone. The more of these you see, the slower things will move."

I nodded, watching an anesthesiologist place a breathing tube down the throat of a middle-aged Dominican man while a nurse attempted to insert an IV.

"Keep an eye on the arrest resident," Baio said and nodded toward the physician at the foot of the bed. "He's in charge. How do you think he's doing?"

"I can't really tell."

I peered around the crowd as someone beat on the man's chest. I thought I heard a rib crack.

"Exactly, you can't tell because he hasn't established that he's in charge. You have to take command of the room."

"Got it." I reached for my pen.

"Don't fucking write this down. Just watch."

The arrest resident began to address the room.

"Speak up," Baio shouted.

The resident's voice rose.

"Second, you have to find out what happened," Baio continued. "First thing you ask is: Did someone witness the arrest? If someone was there to say 'I saw this guy swallow a marble' you've got your answer." Blood splattered near my feet; placing an IV in this man was proving to be difficult. "You know more than you think you do."

It was the second time I'd heard that this morning. "This is getting messy," I whispered back. After a month in the CCU, the sight of blood flying across a room didn't freak me out, but this still seemed like a lot. It was enough to fill a small coffee cup. If I'd seen it in a movie or on television a few months ago, I would've cringed. But it no longer bothered me, and no one else acknowledged the mess coagulating under our shoes. We were a roomful of people comfortable with projectile blood splatter.

"Check out the guy doing chest compressions," Baio said. "How's he doing?"

"Fine, I think."

"Stayin' alive?"

I watched and hummed to myself. "No, he's going too fast."

"Exactly, so if you're in charge you tell him to slow down."

"Should we tell him?"

"No, definitely not. There needs to be one person in charge."

"This is gruesome," I said after blood again splashed in my direction, landing my scrubs, just below the knee.

"How long has it been?" one of the nurses asked me.

"Fourteen minutes," Baio said softly. While I had been dodging blood, he had been quietly keeping time.

"Yikes."

"Always keep an eye on the clock. This is a ghastly funeral."

I looked up at the small black and white clock above the patient's bed. It was the kind my high school had used, and for a brief moment I was transported back to a senior-year classroom, wishing the clock would move more quickly, wishing time would speed up so I could go off to college and start *real* life. Now I was trying to figure out a way to make time slow down. "Should he stop?" I whispered.

Cardiac tamponade was what the more senior doctors in the room suspected, a condition in which blood accumulates around the lining of the heart, leaving it unable to pump properly. The only way to urgently correct it is via pericardiocentesis, a procedure in which a doctor blindly plunges a needle under the patient's rib cage and into the lining of the heart so the fluid can be drained. In this case, it would be done while chest compressions were being performed, making the heart a moving target. Anxious physicians looked back and forth, wondering who should attempt the procedure. It was dangerous. Inserting the needle in an inch too far would pierce the ventricle, almost certainly killing the patient.

"This is not the way you want to go," Baio whispered.

"Should the arrest resident stop?" a nurse quietly asked me. "The guy's been dead for twenty minutes and now they want to stick a needle where?"

"I would," Baio murmured. "I'd stop. But funerals are like weddings—you have to ask if there are any objections before you go through with it."

The pericardiocentesis began and the room fell silent. The physician performing the procedure, a slight Asian man, held the large needle with both hands as it pierced the skin and gradually sunk into the chest. I held my breath as the needle disappeared. The thought of doing this procedure terrified me.

Drops of sweat beaded on the man's wisp of a mustache as the needle submerged deeper. He bit his lip as the needle fully disappeared under the ribs. He pulled back on the syringe, first gently and then with great force, hoping to obtain fluid. But there was nothing. I craned my neck to get a better view.

"I didn't get it," the man said after several minutes and stepped away from the body. Chest compressions continued unabated. A second physician took the needle and prepared to repeat the procedure. A wave of nausea cascaded over me.

"Okay, stop," the arrest resident shouted. "Resuscitation efforts appear futile."

CPR had been attempted for twenty-two minutes.

"Time of death is eleven-fifty-two A.M. Thanks everyone."

And with that, it was over. Nurses and doctors stepped away from the bloodied, lopsided chest and stoically filed out of the room. There were no conversations, no eye contact. Everyone calmly returned to their scut lists and the next task at hand. Baio shook his head and disappeared down a long corridor.

It was the first failed resuscitation that I had witnessed. As the crowd thinned, I moved in and peered over the body. Eventually the room was vacant except for me, the corpse, and another intern. She closed the eyes of the dead man and then softly said, "I would've kept going."

18

The next day I was back on infectious disease rounds, presenting a patient to the team. In contrast to cardiac care unit rounds, this discussion took place around a conference table. Glazed donuts were passed as I spoke.

"So," I concluded, "the patient is doing really well. I actually think he's ready to go home today." David was thirty-four and had walked into our emergency room a few days earlier covered in painful purple and yellow abscesses. A simple staph infection was the cause, but his immune system, ravaged by HIV, was unable to fight it off. It was the third time in the past year that he had come to our hospital with these erupting, rancid skin lesions.

Dr. Chanel ran her hand through her ponytail. "I agree," she said, "but I'd like to get one more set of labs. I'd like to see how the liver is doing before we send him out into the great unknown."

It was 10:15, and morning labs had already been drawn; a phlebotomist would not be on the floor for six more hours. "I'll just draw the labs myself," I announced. I'd come a long way from those first few incompetent days in the CCU. I wasn't ready to do a pericardiocentesis, but I could draw blood.

"Can I join you?" Carleton asked.

"Make it quick," Ashley said, "we've got two waiting for us down in the ED."

I slipped on my white coat, put the dark green stethoscope around my neck, and walked with Carleton across the hall to David's room.

"So exciting," Carleton said. He was far better at faking enthusiasm than I would ever be, which irritated me. My colleagues could sense my hesitancy the moment I walked into the hospital's lobby. But Carleton was the kind of kid who could adapt, who could play the role that was required of him. He was a medical school chameleon; if he needed to be passive—like during psychiatry, where more of the time was spent listening—he could, and if he was called on to be assertive, perhaps during the surgery rotation, he could do that, too. He was the student who would breeze through medical school and residency free from torment, free from anguish. A few years from now he would summer with other beautiful, carefree people in the Hamptons, tossing back cocktails on a private beach.

I tapped on David's door as I pulled it open. A large man with thinning brown hair, he mock-cringed when he saw me.

"Not you again," David said. He shook his head and reached for a magazine.

"Me again," I said cheerily. "This time I have company. I've brought along a medical student, if that's okay."

"This guy tortured me yesterday!" David said with a smile to Carleton. He put the back of his hand to his forehead and added, "I don't know if I'll ever recover."

A day earlier, I'd spent hours lancing every one of his abscesses with a small scalpel and even more time scooping up the pus with gauze. In college, even in medical school, the sight and smell of those abscesses would've made me nauseated, but not anymore. I had been told that every doctor eventually discovers which bodily fluid he or she finds most disturbing, and this realization helps guide the choice of a subspecialty. I didn't mind blood, spit, piss, or pus. I did mind diarrhea, which meant I wasn't destined to become a gastroenterologist.

"Antibiotics weren't going to work," I said. "You know that. I had to open those things up."

"I know, I know," David said, waving his hand dismissively, "you had to do it. But why the CAT scan? That took up my whole afternoon!"

I flashed to Gladstone and shook my head. I was now ordering potentially unnecessary head scans several times a week and neurosurgical consults nearly as frequently. "The good news is you're getting better. The CAT scan was normal and you're going home soon." Even though I suspected that Gladstone was going to be okay, his image haunted me. Whenever I felt like I was starting to get the hang of things, like I was starting to become a real doctor, I was reminded of him and my colossal oversight. More than anything, I was reminded that I needed supervision. Fortunately, Columbia had a structure in place that provided it. But what would happen when I was the supervisor? It was okay to practice defensive medicine for now—I had people like Ashley to tell me when I was being overly cautious—but eventually I'd need to cut the safety net.

"Thank God," David said.

"I'm proud of you for starting the HIV medications. Your numbers were through the roof." I set down the equipment for the blood draw and turned to Carleton.

"You know, it's actually better today to have HIV than diabetes."

"But I have diabetes," David said.

I frowned. "Let's get started."

I knelt down by the side of the bed and again turned to Carleton. "The key to drawing blood is finding a vein. Help yourself out by using a tourniquet." He quickly scribbled on a notepad as I spoke. "Sometimes one isn't available, so I just tie a latex glove around the patient's arm."

"Technically they're latex-free gloves," Carleton said. "Because so many people have latex allergies."

"Right." Fastening the glove, I felt for veins. "His veins aren't great," I said as David wrinkled his brow and looked at his arm. "Have you ever heard of the intern's vein?"

Carleton shook his head. "What's that?"

"It runs along the thumb. Works every time."

Enjoying my new role as teacher, I took out an alcohol swab and wiped down the vein as David looked away. I uncapped the butterfly needle and attached it to a thin plastic tube. The tube was fastened to a small vial and placed in a bucket next to the patient's right leg.

"Before you do a procedure, any procedure," I said, "you should do a time-out. Before you do something to a patient, no matter how trivial, you should bring someone else into the room."

"Got it," he said, writing that down. His copious copying reminded me of myself. But I doubted Carleton ever needed someone to tell him not to write on his hands. He probably already knew about the time-out. He was probably only taking notes to placate me.

I tilted my head at his notepad. "First, confirm that you have the correct patient. Then, double-check that you are, in fact, doing the appropriate procedure to the proper body part."

I confirmed the information and plunged the needle into David's thumb. He reflexively pulled his hand back an inch as blood flowed through the tubing and the vial filled.

"All done," I said a moment later and held up the vial.

With my left hand I withdrew the needle from his thumb and with my right I reached for a Band-Aid. Blood oozed where the needle had been. Not wanting it to drip on the floor, I quickly moved the Band-Aid toward David's thumb.

But the Band-Aid never reached its intended destination. My right hand's path was intercepted by the butterfly needle, and in an instant I had impaled my index finger with the blood-filled needle. I dropped the needle and ripped off my glove. Blood dripped out of my hand as Carleton looked on, mouth agape. Hundreds of thousands of copies of the human immunodeficiency virus had just been injected into my bloodstream.

19

Darkness.

That is all I remember until I heard Carleton's voice.

"Holy shit!" he was shouting, shaking me from a tranquil haze. I dropped to my knees and squeezed the finger, trying to expel the infected blood. My breathing was ragged. I squeezed so hard my finger turned white—I didn't mind if it fell off. "No, don't," Carleton said, inching toward the door. "Don't cause inflammation. It'll draw white cells to the virus and—"

I stared at him blankly. He was an amorphous WASP blob. But he seemed like he knew what to do.

"Sink," he said. "Sink! Wash it out!"

How did Carleton know what to do? Was this a scenario they covered in medical school? I contemplated putting the finger in my mouth. Could I suck the virus out? I looked down at my palm and licked my lips. In my peripheral vision, I caught a glimpse of David. Both of his hands were on his face like Macaulay Culkin in *Home Alone.*

"Wash it out!" Carleton implored.

I felt like I was going to pass out or vomit. Time was somehow simultaneously speeding up and slowing down. I was unable to move, trapped in quicksand just a few feet from the needle, from the blood, and from David. I wanted to scream but I had nothing to say. I wanted to run but I had nowhere to go.

Carleton turned on the faucet and guided my hand toward the stream. We looked at the finger, which was still oozing blood, and looked at each other. His placid face was without a single crease, without a single wrinkle. I wondered what he saw in mine.

I waved my hand under the icy water, and the cold snapped me back into the awful present. Bursting out of the room, I lunged toward a nearby conference room where a group of HIV doctors were known to have lunch. "I'm sorry," I said, frantically throwing the door ajar as six gray heads turned to me. "I just stuck myself. With HIV. Drawing blood I stuck myself."

Dr. Chanel popped up from her chair and gasped, "What?" I cradled my right hand in my left like it was Axel's banana peel. She rushed over and put her hand on my shoulder as the others returned to their conversations. "Are you okay?" she asked slowly.

I wasn't. I couldn't speak. Staring at the finger, I wondered if a scab was forming, sealing the virus inside of me.

"You're going to be okay, Matt," she said deliberately. "You need to go to Employee Health. Okay?" She scanned my eyes to see if this had registered.

"Okay. Where, uh, is that?"

My teeth felt heavy; my lips were numb. I felt like a small child, wanting to run, to disappear, and unable to formulate words.

Chanel grabbed her purse. "Let's go." She put her hand on the small of my back and gave me a gentle nudge out of the conference room. We passed a sheet-white Carleton recounting the event to Ashley, who mouthed "What the?" as we proceeded toward the elevators.

"Who was it?" Dr. Chanel asked. "Which patient?"

The image of Macaulay Culkin's face reentered my consciousness. "David," I mumbled. "It was David."

"Okay," she said, "I'll have to . . . I'll need to make a few phone calls."

A moment later we squeezed into an elevator full of patients and doctors.

"Matisyahu!" a cadre of interns in the back howled, referring to the Jewish rapper and a nickname I had received at a karaoke orientation event. I held up my scut list and shook my head. We were on the ninth floor. Every button had been pressed. On eight I felt a wave of heat rush over me; on seven I got chills. I was going to shit myself.

"You're okay," Chanel whispered.

"Yep." Like a vampire I covered my mouth with the bend of my arm and quietly retched. Sweat gathered around every orifice. The crowd edged away, giving me space to dry-heave.

"Almost there," she said, as the elevator gradually thinned out.

When we arrived at Employee Health, Dr. Chanel removed her hand from my back and spoke to the clinic administrator. The only words I heard were "can't wait," and a moment later I was in a doctor's office, sitting across from a physician from South America who looked like a young Antonio Banderas. Why did everyone at work remind me of an actor? Perhaps it was because hospital life often took on a cinematic quality and I was subconsciously casting a film—one that had just transitioned from drama to tragedy.

Banderas's broad smile and well-coiffed black hair projected an air of genial confidence; he looked like he could be Diego's older brother. He began saying words, but I didn't hear them. There were lots of nods and smiles. I considered his hair gel. He became more animated as I stared at my hands, tracing the creases. Eventually isolated, vexing words from Banderas began to register:

hazard, unfortunate, change, feel, sleepless, fine, support, prophylaxis

It was a new experience to flip back and forth between such unwelcome extremes. One moment I was wholly and vividly present; in the next I was rendered senseless, lost in a fog. I squeezed the finger over and over. First it was to match my surprisingly sluggish heart rate, and then it was to the beat of an eighties song I couldn't get out of my head—"Your Love" by the Outfield. Banderas put a hand on my shoulder and lyrics breezed through my head.

Josie's on a vacation far away . . .

"Matt," he said.

What was the Outfield up to now? I wondered. And who was this man before me and where did he go to medical school? Could I trust him? Was his life, like mine, a series of flashbacks to movies and sitcoms? Did he have hobbies? A mixed martial arts enthusiast, perhaps? Someone who might wear a blouse to a nightclub?

"Matt!" he shouted. "This is important."

I snapped back, as if a train had unexpectedly passed going the opposite direction. "Yes. Yes. What?"

"Matt, do you know if the patient has hep C?"

I shook my head. "I'm sure we checked, but I'm not positive."

Why was he bringing up hepatitis?

"This isn't meant to alarm you." He motioned to a chart on the wall. "But I want you to have all of the information." The chart showed a large syringe with a stream of statistics. Hepatitis C was an order of magnitude more contagious than HIV via needle stick.

"I don't know about the hepatitis," I said. "I'll find out, obviously."

"In addition, Matt, I highly recommend you take the postexposure prophylaxis."

He stepped out and returned a moment later with pills, the same medications I'd spent the morning reciting to myself on the subway, trying to drill their confusing names into my head to impress Ashley. Truvada. Lopinavir. Ritonavir. They sounded like villains in a comic book, each with a bright color and a unique shape. The conversation with Banderas concluded a few minutes later and we shook hands, agreeing to follow up later in the week. He said it was impossible to prognosticate; I might be fine, but I might not. But I didn't want to leave until I had an answer. How could I?

As I stepped out of his office, I imagined the virus frantically swimming like a legion of sperm toward the lymph nodes in my armpits, and from there, racing to my neck and groin. Was HIV starting to replicate inside me? Or was my immune system destroying it? And how would I be able to tell what was happening in my body a day, week, or month from now? Banderas had said there was no way to know; I just had to take the pills and wait. Blood tests with an answer were more than a month away.

I tried to think of something else—anything else—but I couldn't. I imagined a priest reading me my last rites as I writhed in bed. Then an artist's rendering of the human immunodeficiency virus from a textbook appeared. Soon, pill bottles and syringes were dancing across my mind. But the thing that mattered—the scientific realities of viral transmission—remained elusive. The enzymes, the blood cells, the biochemical reactions . . . all of that suddenly seemed hazy. Why couldn't I remember what I needed to remember? I craved clarity but the only thing I could easily picture was a giant question mark blinking atop my head.

Out in the waiting room, Dr. Chanel was standing ramrod straight with her arms behind her back.

"You didn't have to wait for me," I said, touched and relieved that she had.

"Matt," she said, lowering her head, "I spoke to a few people."

"You look worried," I said abruptly. "I mean more worried. What's happening?"

"I spoke to one of our experts. You're going to need to come with me. We can talk on the way."

"I'm sorry?"

She put her hand on my shoulder and her fingernails inadvertently scratched my skin. The tactile sensation cut through my fog. I started to feel uncomfortably present again. "You are going to be okay, but things are a bit more complicated than we realized." Pure, unalloyed fear coursed through me. "Whatever he just gave you for postexposure HIV prophylaxis is insufficient. David has such a highly resistant strain of HIV that you're going to need an extensive regimen of medications."

Her lips went on moving, but I heard nothing. My thoughts turned to the handful of facts I'd learned about HIV in medical school.

Needle sticks were rare, but they happened. Someone did a study and found that of six thousand pricks with HIV-positive blood, the virus was transmitted twenty times. Those were decent odds, but far from perfect. I thought of myself as number twenty-one, which was my old baseball number. I pictured a jersey, a scarlet letter of sorts, with the virus on the front and my name on the back, announcing to the world that I'd contracted a deadly disease through my own incompetence.

I wasn't sure how long Dr. Chanel spoke or how far we walked, but my sensorium cleared when we hit the waiting room of the Columbia outpatient HIV clinic. A handful of men and women were reading magazines and chatting on cell phones, not unlike any ordinary waiting room. What I knew about this patient population had largely come from more senior residents. Based on their salacious anecdotes, I had expected the AIDS clinic waiting room to look like something out of a zombie movie, with drug addicts and the mentally ill shouting and spitting at one another. But these were just regular people—people with families and jobs and pets and credit card bills—who were trying to coexist with a virus. And I was now possibly one of them.

"Come to my office," Dr. Chanel said. "This way."

As we walked down that interminable hallway, time slowed down, just as Baio had said it did for Michael Jordan when he was in the zone. But this felt like the Twilight Zone.

"Take a seat," Dr. Chanel said.

I looked out of her office window. A storm was gathering. My body tingled as the enormity of the moment finally set in. *I might have just given myself HIV. Because of a mistake.* A second's carelessness and I had possibly altered the trajectory of my life. I might have to travel with pill bottles. I might become sickly. I could die. And drawing David's blood wasn't even my responsibility. I had *volunteered*.

Suddenly I was on fire. Rage rippled through my entire body like a shock wave. I looked into Dr. Chanel's aqua eyes and screamed, "Fuck!"

She stared right back at me, unflinchingly holding my gaze.

"I can't fucking believe this! Fuck!" I wanted to hit something as a slew of compound, unimaginative curse words rushed out of me. I wanted to flip over Chanel's desk and break a window. I wanted to channel all of my rage into something else, some other object that was not me. If I broke a window, the shards of glass would also be implicated in this ordeal. I would have something else to blame, something other than my own incompetence. I screamed again. It sounded like a bullhorn, low-pitched and distorted. I imagined the sound waves smacking into the concrete walls of her small office.

Never could I have imagined behaving this way in front of a senior physician, but here I was, scared and unhinged. I felt like I'd just climbed up ten flights of stairs and been kicked in the face. Eventually I paused to catch my breath, aware that I had rather successfully transitioned from the first stage of grief (denial) to the second (anger). Chanel, to her credit, was unfazed. A few hours ago she had been the teacher and I the student. Now she was the doctor; I was the patient.

"Okay, Matt," she said calmly, "you're going to need to be on several medications. Some are once a day, some are twice a day, and one is three times a day. One needs to be refrigerated. I will write you the prescriptions after we go over the side effects, which can be significant."

I had heard her say these very words to the young woman on rounds, the patient who sobbed after Ariel gave her the new diagnosis of HIV. I was thankful that a roomful of medical students and young doctors wasn't here to watch me. I wasn't handling this well. I wanted privacy. I wanted to disappear. I couldn't imagine dealing with this in front of a roomful of strangers. "I'm ready," I said. I wasn't ready. But there was nothing else to say.

I'd often wondered, Why don't HIV patients just take their damn meds? It was something we encountered surprisingly often, and it didn't make sense to me. Even if the side effects were awful, taking the pills was still better than the lethal alternative. Most patients understood the consequences of going off their meds, but many did anyway, and I rarely got a straight answer when I asked why. To skip even one dose seemed incomprehensible to me. Why even think about avoiding something that could save your life?

I was about to find out.

20

After leaving Dr. Chanel's office, I walked out in front of the hospital and took a seat on an unoccupied bench. The thick air was hot and sticky; it was about to rain. I put my head in my hands and began trying to process everything that had just happened. My throbbing eyes were moist, but not from tears. It was as if all of the tiny blood vessels in my eyes had popped and were now slowly leaking onto my eyelids. Dried saliva was caked on the sides of my mouth, and my hair felt like it was standing on end. If anyone had looked like a zombie in the AIDS clinic waiting room, it was me.

I thought of Heather. What would she say? Intuition told me it would be something supportive, although this scenario was so unusual I couldn't be sure. I knew she was asleep, recovering from a thirty-hour shift in the ICU, so I opted not to call her. This conversation would need to be had in person. I looked down at my forearms and imagined the skin covered in abscesses, just like David's. I pulled out my cell phone and scrolled through my contacts. Who should I call? Was this something I could mass-text?

Crazy needle stick at work. HIV scare. I'll be fine. LOL

Probably not. I was suddenly hungry but the thought of actual food made me queasy. I wanted privacy but I didn't. I wanted to blame someone but I couldn't. I closed my phone and my eyes and tried to drown my fear in more facts from medical school. Needle sticks really weren't that uncommon; there had been close to a million in the United States alone, and the people who jabbed themselves tended to be unlucky, not incompetent. My episode with David was an accident, a hazard of the job. A blip. A, dare I say, rite of passage? Maybe something similar had happened to the Badass.

I stood up and made my way toward the falafel cart.

A light rain began to fall as I placed my order. While the vendor drizzled white sauce and hot sauce on the cubes of chicken, my sense of comfort ebbed. There might be a lot of needle sticks, sure, but they were rarely with HIV-positive blood and they were rarely in patients with such a large amount of the virus swimming through their blood vessels. David's blood had hundreds of thousands of copies of HIV in every drop, and for that reason Banderas had classified my stick as high-risk. So it wasn't fair to compare my situation to the average jab, and it wasn't fair to suggest that the Badass had gone through something similar—he was probably an intern before AIDS was even a thing.

I ate half of my falafel and threw out the rest. Part of me was anxious to return to the infectious disease wing—my unexpected absence would put a strain on my fellow interns—but Dr. Chanel had forbidden it. She was coordinating my treatment regimen with the pharmacy and said she'd text-page me as soon as the pills were ready. I took shelter under an awning and waited. Again I pulled out my phone, but I knew I wasn't going to use it. I squeezed it in my right hand as I wiped my eyes with my left, inadvertently introducing hot sauce into my cornea. An occasional gust of wind blew the warm rain onto my skin, like a backyard sprinkler. As the drops of water accumulated on my hands and on my arms, I again envisioned the droplets transforming into hundreds and then thousands of tiny purple pus bubbles. I reached into my back pocket, pulled out the rumpled toilet paper the devastated young woman had waved away, and dabbed my moist eyes.

Eventually the text page from Chanel arrived. I walked across the street to the pharmacy and handed an Indian man the handwritten prescriptions. After I gave him my full name and date of birth, I wanted to say something else, something like "I don't actually have HIV. This is all precautionary. You agree, right?" But I said nothing and waited.

Twenty minutes later I was on the southbound 1 train headed home with a large plastic bag containing all of my new medications. There were eleven pill bottles in all, including medications to prevent nausea and vomiting. Head in hands, I wondered what to say to Heather. I had to tell her, but how? And how would I respond if the shoe were on the other foot? I'd received frantic calls from college friends after "the condom broke," but this was something altogether different. Heather and I had made a point of not talking about work at home, but that was about to end.

"Excuse me, ladies and gentlemen!" someone yelled. It was Ali, wearing suspenders and a top hat. My spiritual healer had returned. He headed in my direction and attempted to hand me another business card, but I waved him away. I didn't want to see him or anyone. I didn't want to touch anyone. And I didn't want to tell anyone. I wanted to be completely alone and I wanted an answer. Did I have HIV or not? Banderas said I wouldn't know for weeks. If the virus didn't destroy me, the uncertainty might.

Emerging from the dank subway at Seventy-Ninth Street and walking toward my soot-stained building, I started examining the bottles of various pills Dr. Chanel had prescribed—ritonavir, lopinavir, tenofovir, darunavir, raltegravir. More comic book characters, all with extensive side effects profiles. Darunavir looked a bit like a football, burnt orange and oval-shaped, while ritonavir was an enormous pale capsule, a meal in a pill that an astronaut might carry. As I twisted the various pill bottles between my thumb and forefinger, I wondered if the medication causing diarrhea would be balanced out by the one inducing constipation.

When I passed a stationery store, I thought of Peter Lundquist and the heart he had drawn on his legal pad, the broken one without any names in it. The one that had brought me to tears. If I couldn't keep it together that afternoon sitting with Denise and Peter, how was I going to deal with this? It was easily the most wrenching thing that had ever happened to me, the kind of thing you heard about happening to other people that made you thankful it wasn't you. This wasn't like waiting for some STD result after a drunken night out; this was a high-risk, life-threatening screwup that could potentially affect everyone I cared about and even those I didn't. For the last month I had watched people in the hospital on the brink of death, but the stakes were always theirs, not mine. I wasn't sure I was up to even waiting to find out my results. And if it turned out I had contracted HIV . . . well, I certainly wasn't ready to think about that version of my future.

"Mr. Matt," the doorman bellowed as I entered the lobby. "How goes it?"

I quickly stuffed the pills back in the bag and gave him a salute. "Terrific."

As I waited for the elevator, my thoughts moved elsewhere. Could I have kids with HIV? Or would the act of conception put Heather at too great a risk? Fuck, I should know this. My mind wasn't working properly. Suddenly I wasn't so sure I knew how Heather was going to respond.

I started running through opening lines to say to her.

So, funny thing happened today at work . . .
Guess who gets to start using condoms again!
I might have AIDS and I would understand if you want to leave me.

I quietly unlocked the door and entered the bedroom. I gave her a light shake, but she was fast asleep. Maybe this could wait. I was terrified of telling her and was looking for an excuse to buy more time. I backed out of the room, but as I was closing the door Heather opened her eyes.

"What?" she asked, wiping sleep from her eyes. "What are you doing home?"

I smiled uncomfortably; words jumped out:

careful understand needle nightmare awful explain Carleton viral sorry

"Holy shit," she said, throwing the blankets onto the floor. "Are you okay?" She bolted out of bed and stood just a few inches from me. "Are you okay?"

She hadn't yet touched me. I wondered if she would. "I had an HIV-positive needle stick this afternoon. I was drawing blood and it just happened."

"Oh my god." She threw her arms around me and said, "Whatever happens, I want you to know that I'm here."

"I don't know exactly how it happened but I just jabbed the fucking thing. I don't know if I blacked out or what."

"Whatever happens," she said, grabbing me more tightly, "I'm here. I'm not going anywhere." I pulled back to look at her face. "I love you," she said, giving me another hug. "I love you. Period."

I stood dumbfounded. It was the most wonderful thing anyone had ever said to me. I reached for the bag of meds, about to show her my new reality, but thought better of it. She gave me another hug, and moments later we crawled into bed and I fell asleep with my hand locked in hers, like Denise and Peter.

I was unceremoniously awoken hours later by an urgent need to move my bowels. Stool vanity cast aside, I was curious to see if my excrement could give me an early indication of my viral status. Could I detect a subtle difference or was I being ridiculous? I wasn't sure.

I thought of my friends and what they would say. But before I contacted them I needed to speak to my mother and father. I'd counseled patients on how to disclose an HIV diagnosis to partners but not parents. A few minutes later I had them both on the phone. A childhood spent watching TBS and Lifetime had taught me what to say next.

"Mom . . . Dad . . . are you sitting down?" I asked solemnly. "Because I'm afraid I have some bad news."

I imagined them on separate phones, just a few feet away from each other in their living room, raising their eyebrows.

"I was drawing blood today and I stuck myself." Silence. "I injected myself with HIV. Several hundred thousand—"

I paused. It occurred to me that my calculation was off—it was impossible to know just how many copies of HIV had been thrust into my finger. I didn't remember David's most recent lab results, and the number might be much higher than that. My parents started speaking, but I only caught fragments.

oh my love you safe when will why would job come home love walk away

My thoughts were somewhere else, trying to remember David's exact HIV viral load. Wasn't it closer to a million? Did it really matter? I returned to my parents.

"It's been a nightmare, obviously," I said.

"You know, Matty," my dad said, his voice rising slightly, "I hate to say it, but this never would've happened if you were a dermatologist!"

It was one of the long-running gags between us and it always made me laugh; insulation from the vagaries of life was only a skin biopsy away. After some obligatory, mutual reassurance, I hung up the phone and crawled back into bed.

21

The next morning I caught my reflection in the bedroom window—my face was droopy and distorted like a Dalí painting—as dozens of numbers whizzed through my head. I had spent the predawn hours devouring research about HIV transmission, hoping that by precisely calculating my risk, I could establish statistical boundaries and somehow contain the nightmare. But the numbers only reinforced the reality of my situation; some unlucky souls were going to contract the virus after a needle stick and I might be one of them. I just had to take my pills, cross my fingers, and wait.

I auditioned various brave faces as I shaved. What if I cut myself? Would HIV-infected blood drip into the sink? I closed my eyes and put down the razor. Now that abject fear had begun to recede, a new, equally terrible feeling was emerging to join it: embarrassment. The idea of walking back into the hospital seemed excruciating. How was I going to face David? Or Ashley? I was a liability, a danger to myself and those around me. How could Ariel and Lalitha and Meghan trust me to do my job? How was I ever going to face all of those AIDS patients—the ones who were disintegrating before my eyes? What were the odds they'd trust a doctor careless enough to accidentally join their fate?

And that was just today. More worrying was what it might do to my reputation and career progress in the long term. Everyone in my intern group felt a pressure, spoken or not, to improve every day—to make diagnoses more quickly, to write notes more adeptly, and to know more about our patients and their illnesses than anyone else in the hospital. We did this by toiling behind the scenes, staying late to talk with a patient's family or coming in early to read up on an obscure disease, and in many cases, we did this by quietly violating strict work hour regulations. No one knew about these violations because we didn't formally punch in and out; we just stayed until the work was done. And the work was never done. Anonymity ultimately meant better care for our patients because we could bend the rules, and I feared that my needle stick would shatter my anonymity; I would become *that guy*, someone people knew about, someone to keep tabs on, and I would not be the only victim of my mistake.

I considered how far word of my needle stick might have traveled in our insular hospital world. Although we didn't have much time to socialize, we had time to gossip. I knew who was screwing, who was pregnant, and who was trying to become pregnant. It was quite easy to attain vast sums of secondhand knowledge of questionable veracity about colleagues I'd never actually spoken to. I could only imagine what would be said about me. How would Ashley relay it? How would Carleton describe it?

What had he said after I was whisked away to meet Banderas? Did the calm, collected medical student describe the incident in detail to his classmates? Did he say I handled the situation well or did he acknowledge the truth—that I was scared and increasingly unable to function as the implications of my mistake set in? And why did I care? The incident was over, there was nothing to do but move forward and tackle the matrix of assignments that was about to unfold. Of course I cared.

I carefully laid out all of the HIV medications on the kitchen table, popping six in quick succession, followed by a glass of water and a handful of cornflakes. The remaining pills I packed in a Ziploc bag and stuffed in the front pocket of my white coat for later. I wasn't technically required to go back to work—supervisors made it clear that I could come back to work when I was ready—but I didn't want to let down my peers. Interns were spread so thin to begin with; sulking at home would only make things worse and perhaps create the perception that I was not a team player. Plus, the fact was that in spite of the psychological blow, there was nothing actually wrong with me. I had to get back to work.

I spent the subway ride to the hospital flipping through *Heart Disease for Dummies* as a mariachi band bounced from one car to the next, but I couldn't focus. I closed the pages and shut my eyes until I arrived at 168th Street.

Entering the hospital, I slipped on my white coat and put my hand in my pocket, rolling the pills through my fingers. The first recognizable face I encountered was that of Benny, who was standing next to a vending machine with a large grin.

"How you doing, big man?" he asked. "You good?"

"Hi, uh, Benny." He was undoubtedly the only patient in the CCU capable of taking a stroll to the vending machines.

He held up a Snickers and giggled. "Don't tell."

He shouldn't be eating that, I thought. "I won't."

"You good?" he asked again, extending a fist. Doctors, nurses, and patients buzzed around us. Some peered into cell phones, others at scut lists. I didn't recognize a single face.

"Well . . ."

"You look a little ashy," Benny said.

Benny, by contrast, looked as well as I'd ever seen him. He was wearing a blue Giants sweatshirt and gray sweatpants and had just finished another session on the stationary bicycle. His enthusiasm for the new NFL season, I soon discovered, was mitigated by his frustration that one of his daughters had been misbehaving at home. I tried to imagine what it must be like for that girl, to miss her father, to tell friends that the old man's not around because he's waiting in the hospital for a heart transplant that might not ever come.

I noticed a small gauze pad near Benny's neck where a large IV had been removed. It reminded me that the man wasn't simply idly waiting, he was constantly undergoing blood tests, MRIs, CAT scans, and X-rays while receiving all sorts of powerful, potentially toxic medications. But to what end? In many ways, Benny reminded me of an intern: smiling on the outside, tortured on the inside.

"Matisyahu!" a passing intern shouted. I gave a small nod and looked into the vending machine for Doritos. My appetite momentarily appeared stronger than my resolve. Thoughts of the needle caused my index finger to throb; I wondered if I should cover the finger with a Band-Aid or if that would only draw attention to the site.

"I'm still waiting," Benny said.

"I figured," I said, referring to his impending heart transplant. "How much longer do they expect?"

He shook his head. "Still waiting for you to tell me you're good." He pointed the Snickers at me like it was a pistol. "Gonna make me ask again?"

I pounded his fist and smiled. "I'm good."

He looked at me askance. "Yeah?"

"Yeah. Took your advice . . . slowed things down, not in such a hurry." I hadn't rushed that blood draw, had I? My mind jumped back to the needle stick, as it had every hour or so since it happened, and again I tried to figure out what went wrong. My mind leapt ahead a few years, to a time when I was just another patient in the HIV clinic. One who couldn't drink alcohol because of the hepatotoxic side effects of ritonavir, one who might need weekly dialysis because of the dangerous side effects of tenofovir, which I learned could tear up the kidneys. I imagined myself on a waiting list, just like Benny, hoping for a new organ after my own had been eaten away by HIV.

"Whatever it is, Matt, you'll get through it."

"I'm good!" I insisted, giving him another fist pound. "What's new in the CCU?"

"Reading a good book," he said. "*Sick Girl,* about a heart transplant."

"Haven't read it."

"And"—he winked—"it's Bad Girls Week on *Judge Joe Brown.*"

A moment later my pager went off: PATIENT WITH ILLICIT ITEMS IN HER BUST. PLEASE EVALUATE.

"Popular," he said, looking beyond me to a small boy holding a balloon. "Stay positive, friend."

"I will," I said. "Gotta run."

"Gotta walk," he said, taking one last bite of the candy bar.

I looked at the pager again, shaking my head at the impending search and seizure, and softly said, "Amazing things . . ."

"They're happening," Benny said, pointing at the slick, off-white floor, "right here."

Exiting the elevator a few minutes later, I bumped into Ashley. "Question," she said, pointing at my belly.

My knees buckled. What was she going to say about the incident? I was in no mood to relive the moment with her or be admonished for my sloppiness. "What's up?" I asked nervously.

"Need your opinion."

"Of course."

"Would you rather marry someone who cheats on you one time or marry an alcoholic?"

She smiled, and a wave of relief washed over me. "Love this question."

"So do I."

We had occasionally batted this around in medical school. The consensus was to marry the person who cheats, but Heather and I had both initially said alcoholic.

"I'd go with the alcoholic," I said to Ashley. "No question."

She shook her head. "No way!"

I shrugged. "Maybe I have trust issues."

"Have you ever lived with an alcoholic?"

"No."

"Then you can't answer the question."

I smiled. "Let me amend my answer. I cannot answer your question because I have never lived with an alcoholic."

Her pager buzzed and she shook her head. "See you in rounds, pal. You're good."

That stupid interaction with her glorious cheekbones was just what I'd needed. She'd treated me like nothing had happened. I didn't have to feel embarrassed; I didn't have to defend actions or offer some lame excuse. Perhaps things would unfold differently in the next few days, but for now, Ashley had tacitly let me know that I'd be able to focus on being a good doctor and not worry about what everyone around me might think.

"P.S.," Ashley said, skipping away, "I think you broke Carleton. Holy shit balls!"

22

I glanced at my scut and tried to prioritize. My instinct told me that the only way I'd make it through the next six weeks without tearing my hair out from worry would be to throw myself even deeper into the job, to focus on the patients. Even this, however, presented a major problem: I was about to spend a month immersed in the world of HIV/AIDS patients while waiting to find out if I was going to become one of them. Each interaction offered a possible mirror into a future I was hoping desperately to avoid.

Based on my experience with David, I feared that I would ultimately internalize all of my patients' symptoms—that an AIDS rash would become *my* rash, that the intractable abdominal discomfort would become my pain, and that the misanthropy, which was pervasive on the HIV floor, would become mine, too. Many felt uncared for, unloved, as though life had passed them by because of the stigma of their illness. It terrified me to think I might join this group. Insomuch as I had a plan, it was to do whatever I could to improve my patients' health so that their condition might karmically rub off on my own.

First up on the scut list was the patient with the possible breast paraphernalia. I noticed that there was no information yet available on her. She had been admitted overnight and would be presented on rounds later in the morning. I trudged up the stairs and braced myself as I approached her room. It's possible I was too close to this disease to treat it effectively.

"Hello?" I said, slowly opening the door.

"Hello," replied a soft, deep voice. I found myself looking at a middle-aged black woman weighing no more than eighty pounds. She was wearing baggy scrub pants and a white T-shirt and had dozens of smooth bumps on her forehead and cheeks that recalled a textbook image of smallpox, a disease that had been eradicated in 1979, the year before I was born. They were different from the abscesses I'd seen on David—the sores didn't appear to be filled with pus. They seemed like they'd been on her face for a long time and weren't going anywhere anytime soon. What could it be? Measles? Chicken pox? Acne? She turned her head away from the door. "Who is it?"

"Dr. McCarthy," I said. "I heard there was some excitement in here."

"No excitement," she said, still looking away.

"One of the nurses paged me," I said, pausing to consider the proper phrasing, "because there was an item found in your blouse."

"I'm not wearing a blouse."

She wasn't. "In your bra."

"I'm not wearing a bra."

I was miffed and let out a quick sigh. "I was paged because a nurse found something and wanted me to have a look."

"Have a look," she said, turning to me. I started quietly as we made eye contact. Her eyeballs were almost completely whited out, as if snow had accumulated on the sidewalk and no one had bothered to shovel it away. What could cause that? A few tumbleweeds drifted across the serene vista that was my uncluttered mind; my differential diagnosis consisted solely of glaucoma. Moranis could probably name thirty things that would cause her eyes to look like that.

"What am I looking at?" I asked.

"There," she said, pointing to a stack of clothes, "probably over there." She motioned to the corner of the room, which meant she might have some vision. I again looked into her eyes, hoping to find some clue that would tie everything together, that would explain the bumps and the eyes and the HIV, but I was stumped. I picked up a red and black plaid shirt and a pair of shorts. In the breast pocket of the shirt was a small plastic bag containing something resembling marijuana.

"It's medicinal," she said flatly.

"Is it?" I asked with optimism.

"Yes."

"For what?"

She scoffed. "I'm blind. I'm homeless. I have AIDS. Want me to keep going?"

"What's it for . . . specifically?"

I was fairly certain that medicinal marijuana wasn't legal in the state of New York. Were there exceptions for AIDS patients? I should know this. "I want to believe you."

"Then believe me."

"Do you have a prescription for it?"

She leaned back. "And if I don't?"

I wrinkled my brow. "I'm not sure. I guess I'll have to . . . I'll . . ."

She shook her head. "Why are you doing this to me?"

I looked at the green leaves in the plastic bag and sighed again. "You know I have to report this."

The words sounded funny coming out of my mouth. Did I need to report this? I wasn't sure. In medical school I had tended to a lot of admitted drug users, but none of them had brought the material into the hospital. This seemed more like a job for security than for an intern.

"You don't have to." She flashed a handful of yellow-brown teeth. "Please. Please don't." There was a note of desperation in her voice, and I genuinely wasn't sure what I should do. Was I just another guy trying to make her life more difficult? Or was I a responsible intern, appropriately seizing and reporting banned items? And anyway, what was the point of taking away a blind, homeless AIDS patient's marijuana? It seemed borderline cruel. Where did this fall on the spectrum of *Do no harm*?

I made a snap decision to hide behind the lab coat. "I hate to use this phrase, but I'm just doing my job."

"Come here," she said, waving me toward her. "Come here. Close."

"We have rounds," I said, planning an escape route and then aborting it as Benny's advice flashed through my mind. If there was one thing that Benny had impressed upon me, it was the importance of giving patients my time and my full attention. It was the same thing Jim O'Connell had preached. Since my talk with Benny and then catching myself in the act of backing away from Peter Lundquist, I had willed myself to be more present with my patients. Even so, it was exceedingly difficult to do. Interns were needed in six places at once, and the pager never stopped buzzing. The day was highly scheduled, with meetings and rounds and note-writing, but it was also incredibly unpredictable. Chatting with a patient often seemed like a discretionary activity, even when it wasn't.

I took off my white coat and sat at the edge of the bed.

"What's your name?" she said.

"Dr. McCarthy. Matt McCarthy."

"Matt McCarthy . . . M and M."

"M and M, just like the candy."

"And the rapper. Eminem."

"Indeed," I said. And just like the Morbidity and Mortality conference, I thought. "What should I call you? Your first name or—"

"Call me Dre," she said, giggling to herself. "You're Em and I'm Dre."

"Excellent."

She shook her head. "So why do you want to snitch on me?"

I almost snorted. She had found her way right to the heart of my dilemma. "I don't want to. What am I supposed to do?"

Before I knew what was happening, she'd reached out her hands and put them on my face. One covered my left eye and the other pressed into my right cheek. The move left me frozen. No one had ever done something like this to me before. Her moist, callused hands moved across my face, briefly pausing on my eyebrows and lips. She smelled of lotion, something lavender. I hoped that whatever had caused the bumps on her face wasn't contagious. The needle stick popped into my mind and I pushed it out. "I can tell you're conflicted," she said, sounding like a late-night television fortune-teller. "I can tell."

"I'm not actually conflicted," I said, leaning back slightly.

"Didn't they teach you that the patient is always right?"

I laughed and she grabbed my hands, putting them on her face. She had innumerable keloid scars on her ears from piercings gone awry. What looked like little mushrooms on her earlobes were actually the results of skin healing improperly. I had seen it often in medical school and knew they weren't contagious. But by the sheer number of mushrooms, I doubted that she had been informed of her condition and had tried to pierce the ears over and over again, which only made the condition worse. I wondered what she knew of her other medical conditions. Were we connecting here? In the hospital movie in my mind, touching her face would help me to know her in some unique, previously unavailable way. But in reality, it didn't. It only made me feel bad for her. It made me want to know more about her condition and how I could help her get better.

"I think the saying is that the *customer* is always—"

At that moment, as our hands were on each other's faces, Ashley had the good fortune to enter the room. "I was looking for my intern," she said, looking up from her pager. "I think he— *What the fuuuuck?*"

Stunned by the scene before her, she did a pirouette and exited the room in one motion as I dropped my hands. I got up, squeezed the small bag of marijuana in my palm, and straightened my coat. "You'll see me again."

"No snitchin'!" Dre said as I closed the door. "Don't do it, Em!"

As I walked toward the nurses' station, a number of thoughts buzzed through my head. I'd just been pawed by a legally blind AIDS patient and was suddenly carrying about a hundred dollars' worth of weed in my white coat. This wasn't how Jim O'Connell would do things. I couldn't imagine him seizing drugs from one of his patients. But I also thought that Jim might have appreciated some aspects of the exchange. Dre wasn't the typical patient. Not least because of the mutual face massage, but also because of the undercurrent of humor in our conversation. This was the kind of patient I could see him reaching, the type he'd spend extra time with to make a connection. Why? What was it about her? I wasn't entirely sure. I often had trouble predicting which patients would receive extra attention from Jim, but I felt confident that Dre would've been one of them.

I dropped the bag on the large wooden table and took a seat next to Ashley. "I had to confiscate this."

"That's some freaky shit, man," she said, laughing. "I said you were the eyes and I was the brain. Clearly you're also the hands."

23

Rounds started a few minutes later. Donuts were passed around, and my ears pricked up when the overnight intern, Lalitha, presented Dre's case.

"A congenital infection left her without vision before she reached adolescence," Lalitha said, as she tied her dark hair into a ponytail. "She was infected with HIV a decade ago and since then has lived a life of almost implausible hardship, bouncing from one abusive relationship to the next, rarely living at the same address for three consecutive months." Dre had not taken any of her pills for months and, based on some preliminary laboratory information and physical exam findings, appeared to have neurosyphilis, a severe neurologic complication of untreated syphilis. The disease can cause the brain to see and hear all kinds of unusual things—from mysterious voices to symphonies—and the diagnosis is made via spinal tap, which Dre was refusing.

Dre had provided Lalitha with some of her medical history but not all. Large gaps existed regarding the way she'd contracted HIV, what infections she'd encountered, and what medications she was currently taking. Dre had informed the overnight team that the information would be provided on a need-to-know basis because she wasn't convinced that all of the intrusive medical questions were necessary. And she was refusing HIV medications, which made me want to know more about her. Why would someone turn down potentially lifesaving treatment?

I thought about how neurotic I'd become after acquiring my own set of pill bottles. I didn't want people at work to know how or when I was taking my medications, or what the pills were doing to my insides. Every time I swallowed a pill, it felt like I was ingesting a tiny hand grenade, one that would explode when I least expected it, leaving me doubled over in abdominal pain or rushing to the bathroom to shit my brains out. I didn't want other doctors to know that I occasionally excused myself from rounds because I thought I was going to vomit, or that my bowel movements fluoresced, because I didn't want to be judged. Perhaps Dre thought she would be judged, too. Perhaps she just wanted to be left alone.

There was something about her, however, that made me think she could be reasoned with. Maybe it was that moment when she'd touched my face, maybe that was her very literal way of reaching out to me. Perhaps I was someone *she* wanted to connect with. My mind started to race with possibilities. If I could engage with her in a way that was comforting, or that she respected, I might be able to get through to her and unlock the details of her medical history the way O'Connell would. Someone needed to; whether she knew it or not, Dre was a very sick woman. Without taking HIV meds she might be dead in months, and if she had neurosyphilis, things could get even more complicated. The more we could find out about her, the better. But that would come from sitting with her, talking with her, getting to know what made her tick. It would not come from reading a textbook or from snitchin'.

"Excellent presentation," Dr. Chanel said when Lalitha had finished. "Anyone have anything to add?"

Ashley glanced at me and put her hands to her face, fighting back laughter.

It was time to snitch. Now that I'd told Ashley, I had no choice. "Yes," I said. "I was called to see the patient this morning because she had something that looked like marijuana in her shirt pocket." Collective nods. "I gave it to the nurse manager."

"Very good," Dr. Chanel said. "Shall we go see the patient?"

Apparently this nugget of information was inconsequential. But how was I to know? I wouldn't tell Dre that I had mentioned the drugs to others. Walking down the ninth-floor hallway, Chanel again put her hand on my lower back. "You doing okay?"

"Hanging in there." This was situationally true but a lie in spirit. I was a throbbing ball of anxiety, having returned to full teeth-grinding mode in the last eighteen hours. Thinking about Dre's dilemma was a useful distraction but hardly a cure. A thousand thoughts threatened to spill out of me in response to Chanel's simple question, but this wasn't the time or the place to be a patient. I was on rounds and we had work to do.

"Let me know if you need Zofran," she said, referring to the powerful antinausea medication. "Expensive, but it works." She gave me a hint of a smile, and I returned it.

"Thank you for getting me through everything," I said softly, recalling the slew of curse words I'd spat at her the day before. I'd spent the first month of my internship standing in awe of Baio, the man who could handle any clinical conundrum, but in Chanel I saw something unique, something I admired just as much. She had functioned as a sounding board, and let me feel comfortable saying or doing anything in her presence. If I wanted to have a meltdown, I could, and I knew she wasn't going to think any less of me.

"I'll let you inform the patient of our plan," she said softly, running her fingers through her side ponytail. A moment later, our team formed a horseshoe around Dre. Heads gradually turned in my direction, and I cleared my throat, wondering how familiar I should be with her in front of the other residents. I had heard such intimate details of her troubled life, but we'd really only exchanged a handful of words and they were all about marijuana.

"Is that you, Em?" she asked.

I blushed at the nickname. "I'm here. With the entire team, actually. Before we get started, would you prefer to be addressed by your first name or last?"

"Just call me Dre," she said.

After summarizing our interpretation of her case, we examined her one by one. Her neck was exceedingly stiff, so rigid and tender she couldn't touch her chin to her chest, and she was mostly numb below her shins. I had hoped to examine her pupils to look for one of the hallmarks of neurosyphilis, but she told me she'd had enough of being prodded and wanted to take a nap.

"The long and the short of it," I said as I put my penlight back into my white coat, "is that we're worried about you. You need a spinal tap." Lalitha had explained this to her overnight, but I wasn't sure how much of it had registered.

"No, thank you," she said, closing her eyes.

"And you need to get back on your HIV meds."

"No. Thank you."

I turned to Dr. Chanel for guidance; she raised her eyebrows as if to say, "Go on."

"You need the test," I said firmly, "and you need the meds." Perhaps it was just a matter of persistence.

"No." She folded her arms and again turned away from me. "Not happenin'."

How could I reach her? Did Dre realize what she was up against? Maybe not. Maybe that was the problem. "You could die. Honestly."

"Fine," she said, "let me."

I opened my mouth, but nothing came out. She had short-circuited my one ironclad logical point. *Let her die?* What was I supposed to say? I could treat her HIV and what appeared to be neurosyphilis, but how was I supposed to treat whatever made her favor dying over taking the pills?

Standing before her, I felt the glare of my colleagues. Chanel must have sensed my cognitive dissonance. She sat down on the edge of the bed. "Can we talk about this later, one-on-one?"

"You can talk," Dre said, "talk all you want."

"Very well," Chanel said. "I'll come back later."

We stepped out of the room and discussed the approach to this difficult patient. Everyone agreed that a multidisciplinary approach would be necessary, incorporating psychiatry, social work, nursing, and potentially a host of other specialists.

As we discussed options, I went over the interaction again and again in my head. Why had my approach foundered? Could what I had said even be described as an approach? All I did was explain the scenario and try to scare her into compliance. I had assumed the specter of death would be enough. It was more than enough for me. In less than a day the pills I was taking had already begun to liquefy my insides, but I'd take pills that rotated my head 180 degrees before I'd give myself over to fate when it came to HIV. If I was going to get through to Dre, I'd have to figure out how she saw things.

The challenges I encountered on the HIV floor were so different from what I'd dealt with in other areas of medicine. There was a right way to do chest compressions, a proper way to adjust a ventilator. Do this and don't do that. The skills I needed on the HIV floor—tact, patience, empathy—were more abstract. But the stakes were just as high; if I failed to acquire these traits, patients could die.

What if something else was going on with Dre, something I'd missed entirely? Maybe there really were voices in her head telling her not to take the pills. Then what? Could we force her to accept treatment? The ethics of medicine were bewildering.

"Tough crowd," Ashley said, patting me on the back.

"Yeah."

"Give it another shot after lunch. She likes you."

"She hides it well."

"I saw the way she let you paw her face." I'd noticed a change in Ashley's demeanor toward me. The drill sergeant act had been cast aside; in its place was someone who was treating me with kid gloves. I couldn't tell if that was a good thing.

We walked back to the conference room and finished rounds. As

Lalitha, who had been up for more than twenty-four hours, presented the next case—flawlessly maintaining the role of exuberant, compassionate, put-together intern—I stared at the small clock on the wall, counting the minutes until I was due for my next dose of comic book villains. I thought of the burnt-orange football and of the astronaut pill. The medications tasted rather bland, except for ritonavir, the sweet one, which was encased in a sugary capsule and tasted like a Flintstones vitamin. I wondered if Dre took any of these pills, or if she'd forgotten what medications she was on and felt embarrassed. I was tempted to leave rounds and show them to her, but I wasn't sure what she'd be able to see. Was it wise to show a legally blind woman a handful of pills and ask if they looked familiar?

As Lalitha began drawing on a marker board, I felt for the pills in the pocket of my white coat, rolling each one back and forth in my fingers, wondering exactly how long they would be a part of my life. It was a mistake to think about my own condition when we still had patients to discuss, but I couldn't help it. Dr. Chanel said I had to take the assortment of medications for a minimum of four weeks but possibly longer. Possibly forever.

"Your luck continues," Ashley said after rounds. "Today is intern report."

I shook my head. "What's that?"

"I hold your pager for an hour while you have lunch with the other interns and vent."

The thought appealed to me, mostly. I had so much I wanted to say and discuss. Were others slogging through internship the way I was? Or were they gliding effortlessly, as I imagined Carleton would. I still hadn't met all of the interns—spending three years in a pod of four would undoubtedly have its benefits, but the isolation also seemed a significant drawback. Of the group I had started the year with, I'd probably spoken to only half. I had shared a beer with only a handful and rarely seen anyone let their guard down. We were all trying to fit in as real doctors while maintaining our pristine, gilded personas. It was exhausting.

"If nothing else," Ashley said, "it's an hour break."

I slipped out of the conference room and headed down a long corridor, feeling my stomach rumble along the way. It was almost time to pop the pills. Replaying my appeals to Dre, I considered new tactics. Good cop? Share my own experience? Beg.

I entered the standing-room-only intern report, where a youngish physician—a chief resident named Dave—stood before a marker board addressing close to forty seated interns. In his left hand was a butterfly needle and in his right was a tourniquet. I scanned the room for familiar faces as I meandered toward the paper plates, soda, and pizza.

"Seven needle sticks already this year," Dave said loudly, adjusting his glasses. "Far too many." A few eyes from the crowd looked in my direction as I took my first bite. "This should really be second nature by now." I felt a swirl of anger when his eyes met mine. This was supposed to be a venting session, not a harangue. "We're going to review the basics of drawing blood today," he went on. "The key to this, as in any procedure, is to focus. You can't be in a hurry and you can't be sloppy. Take pride in your work."

I felt like he was talking directly to me, suggesting that my mishap had something to do with a lack of respect for the profession. But as I processed the words and looked out at the room, I also felt a sense of relief. I wasn't the only one. My colleagues were sticking themselves, too. In theory, we weren't even supposed to draw blood—the hospital hired professional phlebotomists to do that. But if one of them failed to find a vein or was unable to convince a patient that the blood test was necessary, we were called in for mop-up duty. There had been no orientation seminar on how to draw blood, no guidebook or instruction manual. As with so many other things, we had been forced to figure it out on our own.

I scanned the room, looking at each intern's face, searching for a glimpse of discomfort or anguish—a sign that someone else was dealing with the fallout of a needle stick. But what I mostly saw was exhaustion. As the greasy pizza was devoured, I caught several interns surreptitiously tapping their hips, checking for pagers that, for this solitary hour, were not there.

A hand grabbed my arm. It was Ariel. Her tangle of frizzy red hair was now in two pigtails like Pippi Longstocking. "Let's go," she whispered, ushering me out of the room. "Wendy's."

We walked down the hall in silence, finishing our pizza. It was the first real food I'd eaten since the falafel cart. Ariel smiled and gently patted me on the back, like I was a child and she was encouraging me to eat.

Due to our call schedules, I'd spoken to Ariel more on rounds than in private. She knew almost nothing about me and I knew exceedingly little about her, but I suddenly felt like we were old friends; we had shared a lot of experiences as pod mates, enough for her to feel protective of me when intern report promised to be more anxiety-making than calming. I appreciated that she was getting me out of the hospital. "The way I figure it," Ariel said when we stepped into the empty elevator, "you could teach that class."

"Thank you for saving me."

As the elevator plunged toward the lobby, I felt an anger bubbling up inside of me. Sure, there had been six other needle sticks this year, but how many of them had involved HIV-positive blood? How many interns had been handed a sack full of HIV pills to hide in their lockers? How many were worrying if they'd be able to have a child without passing on the virus?

The wave broke as we exited the hospital. "Fuck!" I blurted as we walked down the street together. "I feel like fucking shit! Fuck!"

Rather than ducking my words, Ariel leaned in and intentionally bumped shoulders with me. "Fuck and shit?" she asked. "I hear that's bad."

"Fucking shit." I laughed. "Also bad."

We walked south along Broadway, mostly in silence, and reached Wendy's a few minutes later. "Two double cheeseburgers and two Frosties," I said, assuming my companion was not a vegetarian. I imagined Ariel in her previous life as a consultant, having a steak lunch with clients in midtown, discussing profit margins.

"Still have your appetite, I see."

"Sort of."

"I can't imagine," she said, "what yesterday must have been like."

"I don't really want to talk about it."

"Neither do I," she said as we brought our food to a small booth. We toasted Frosties and reflexively felt for our absent pagers.

"You ever watch *Saved by the Bell*?" I asked, still thinking about Dre's marijuana and my decision to report it.

"Once or twice."

"There's this scene," I said, preparing to quote what was arguably the show's most famous line, "where one of the girls, Jessie Spano, gets hooked on caffeine pills and has a meltdown. She starts crying and screaming *I'm so excited, I'm so excited, I'm so scared.*"

Ariel dipped her pinkie finger into her Frosty and smiled. "Matt, are you having a Jessie Spano moment?"

Ariel was a soft touch; she could shoot the shit with anyone. As the weeks went by, I was discovering that there were two types of interns: those who had gone straight from college to medical school to internship, and those, like Ariel, who had not. The latter group seemed to have a distinct, more comfortable way of interacting with patients. I thought about the way she had delivered the new HIV diagnosis to the young woman. It was a difficult spot to be in, but she'd handled it well. Better than I would have, certainly. Her approach was less frantic, less forced. Perhaps it was simply age and maturity, or maybe it was something else.

As we ate our food, I thought about telling Ariel about the needle stick—as if going through each painstaking detail would help me move on. But the words didn't sound right in my head—it felt like I was seeking pity, or looking to sensationalize a mistake. Ariel wasn't my therapist and she wasn't my doctor.

"You know," I said, looking out of a large window, "this stuff we do all day . . . it's a weird job." She nodded. "It's like it could be a movie. Or a TV show. Or a book."

She grinned.

"And sometimes," I went on, "a lot of the time, actually, I just feel like things aren't clicking."

"I know what you mean."

She had graduated at the top of her class. I wasn't sure if she was just humoring me. "Really?"

"Yeah."

"Sometimes I worry I'm a hazard—to myself, to the patients." I suppose I did want to talk about it. The needle stick had further undermined my self-confidence, and it was eating away at me. I needed to tell someone so I wasn't dealing with it alone. "I don't feel that way all the time, but sometimes I do."

"We could drop you in one of those hazmat bins."

"You think I'd fit?" I asked, raising an eyebrow.

"Matt," she said, putting down her burger, "it was an accident. You heard: seven sticks already."

"And," I said, "I have to wonder, temperamentally, if this job is—"

"Hold that thought," Ariel said as she stood up. "Let's get another round."

We got back in line and reviewed the menu—there was something decadent and mischievous about ignoring medical advice and gorging ourselves on double cheeseburgers and Frosties. I imagined thousands of tiny French fries clogging my arteries.

"I feel like . . ." I considered the proper way to phrase my vague unease. "This sounds silly but . . . I feel like I'm a wall that needs to get painted. And every day a bit of paint gets splattered on me." Ariel grinned. "It's like every time I see a new patient or a new case, a bit of paint gets splattered."

"What color paint are we talking about?" she said, popping a French fry into her mouth, "just so I'm with you."

I looked at the ketchup packets between us. "Red."

Now we both grinned.

"A lot of days," I went on, "I see the same shit—heart failure, pneumonia, blood clots—and the same parts of the wall get painted. But there are these huge blank spots on the canvas. Reading about cases does nothing for me. I fall asleep before I can finish a page. I have to see it in person or it never happened. But what about rare diseases? What'll happen when I'm the attending and I'm confronted with a dying patient and a constellation of symptoms I've never seen before?"

"I feel the same way," Ariel said flatly. "Can't learn medicine from your sofa."

Ariel might have been humoring me—I imagined she had glided through her rotations much in the way that Carleton would—but I doubted it. It felt like she was similarly in search of a way to learn everything about everything.

"And now, of course, I've got other shit on my plate." I shook my head and glanced down at my finger. "I still can't believe it."

"We're all dealing with something."

I waited for her to expand on the thought. I wanted to know what she was dealing with. Had she made mistakes? Been talked down to? Or yelled at? Was she befriending patients like Benny? I hadn't seen any of that, possibly because I was so wrapped up in my own world, just trying to get through each exhausting day.

I waited and waited but Ariel didn't elaborate, and I wasn't sure how much I could push. I wondered if her reticence had more to do with giving me the chance to vent or with keeping her cards close. It would've been the reflexive thing to do. Even intern report, ostensibly a place for new physicians to let their guard down, had turned into a remedial tutorial on the basics of phlebotomy.

Ariel turned her head to look outside. She again felt for her absent pager.

"Anyway," I said, breaking the silence, "I can assure you this damn needle stick is singed into my brain forever. And I will never, ever forget the side effects of HIV meds."

"I bet." She raised her Frosty. "You're going to be okay."

"You think?" *Lie to me,* I wanted to say, *lie to me if you have to.*

"One day this'll be just another splotch of blood on the wall."

"Paint," I said, smiling as I dabbed my right index finger with ketchup. "Let's stick with paint."

Ariel glanced at her watch and we stood up; playtime was over. We had pagers to retrieve and patients to see. And I had a date with a bagful of HIV pills.

24

"My gift to you," Ashley said, handing me my pager ten minutes later. "Thing never stopped buzzing."

"*Gracias.*"

"How was intern report?" she asked.

"Fine," I said. "Listen, I'm gonna give it another shot with Dre." On the walk back from Wendy's I had tried to think more about how to break through to her. I hadn't come up with much, but I felt momentarily invigorated by my lunchtime heart-to-heart with Ariel. "I think what she needs is some tough love." I imagined what Ariel might say to Dre. "Or the opposite. I really have no idea."

"I wanted to talk to you a bit more about her. Something that didn't come up on rounds."

"Of course."

Ashley pulled out a sheet of laboratory data. "Do you think she needs dialysis?"

I scratched my head. "Someone mentioned kidney disease, but I'm not sure she needs dialysis."

"Why not?" She batted her hazel eyes. "Walk me through your thought process."

"It's going to be a short walk."

"Try."

"Her creatinine is almost three," I said, referring to the blood test that reflected kidney function. A normal value hovers around one. "Not great but not horrible."

"Fine."

I recalled the handful of patients I'd taken care of with kidney failure. "Dialysis is usually an emergency."

"Sometimes. But not always."

"Okay. I mean, she looks stable. Sick but stable. I can call and arrange dialysis, certainly."

"When you call, you have to make a case for it." She put her thumb and index finger together and stared deep into my eyes. "The nephrologists are busy and it's a pain in the ass to dialyze someone. You gotta have a leg to stand on. What's your argument?"

"I'd say her kidneys are only marginal and to be on the safe side we should do it."

"Wrong!" She made the sound of a gong. "Never say 'to be on the safe side.' We're in a hospital—that's a given." She took a large swig of her latte. "Remember your med school lectures on dialysis?"

"Vaguely."

"It can all be distilled down to this: A-E-I-O-U." She motioned to my breast pocket, and I pulled out a pen to take notes. "A. Acidosis—is the patient's blood acidic? If so, dialysis. E. Electrolytes. If an electrolyte is severely off—"

She pointed at me.

"Dialysis," I said.

"Good. I. Intoxication—did the patient ingest something toxic like moonshine or overdose on something like lithium?"

Dialysis had always confused the shit out of me. Was it really this straightforward?

"O. Overload. Is there fluid overload—too much liquid on the lungs?"

Her approach on this recalled Baio's, and I knew I wouldn't forget it. The truth is that complex decisions are often made using simple mnemonics. Linguistic shorthand wasn't encouraged at Harvard—information needed to be mastered before it could be abbreviated—but

Ashley had just simplified a series of baffling medical school lectures on dialysis into a mouthful of vowels.

My pager went off in mid-scribble. I glanced down at it.

THE GREAT MUSTACHE RACE—YOU IN?

I tilted the pager out of Ashley's line of view. "U. Uremia," she said quickly, "and that's it. A-E-I-O-U."

"Wow."

"Next year, the Ash Safety Net disappears," she said, putting a warm hand on my shoulder, "and the Republicans take over. You're on your own. That said, you're doing a good job. Just try to relax a bit."

I no longer felt like deadweight, and she no longer seemed like an annoyed babysitter. Was it because of the needle stick? Or something else? She knew I stayed late and arrived early, that I cared deeply about my job and that I wanted to get better at being a doctor. Perhaps I had earned her respect and she felt invested in me as a member of her team. Or maybe she just felt bad for me. I wanted to know what had changed, but I couldn't figure out how to ask.

"All right," I said, standing up, "thanks for that mnemonic. Time to joust with Dre."

"Good luck."

"Any final words of wisdom?"

She stood up and clasped her hands together. "Get on your knees, Matt, and grovel."

"Seriously?"

"I don't know. What would *you* want to hear?"

As Ashley scuttled away, I stared at the Impressionist seascape hanging on the wall and racked my brain. How had I been talked into unsavory things in the past? Fear, deceit, alcohol, and money came to mind— tactics that weren't appropriate here. I'd jumped at the offer of HIV medications, but that scenario wasn't really applicable either. My biggest fear was skydiving. How could someone talk me into jumping out of an airplane? They couldn't. I wouldn't even consider doing it. What would Jim say to Dre? Or Baio?

I had a new tactic in mind, one that was risky and would potentially leave me exposed, but I had a hunch it might work and I was running out of options. I simultaneously knocked and opened the door to Dre's room a few minutes later. "That you, Em?" she asked.

"How do you always know it's me?"

"Smell," she said, leaning back in bed.

"Seriously? What smell?" I glanced at my armpits.

"I'm playin'! It was just a hunch."

I sat on the edge of the bed—doing so really did force me to listen. "So," I said, taking her soft left hand in mine, "you were about to say you're ready to get back on the meds."

She pulled her hand back slightly, but I didn't let go. "Nope."

"Please."

"No, thank you."

I hadn't yet asked her what she was so afraid of. Death? That couldn't be it. Without the medications, she would die. Sure, I now found myself dealing with diarrhea so aggressive it occasionally left bloodstains on the toilet paper, but there was no other option. I tried to put myself in her shoes, but where did that leave me? In her position I'd take the pills. "Help me understand what's going on."

"I'm impervious to your advances, Em."

I returned to my own fear. No amount of begging or reasoning could get me to strap on a parachute and take that leap. The only way I'd do it is if you pinned me down against my will and shoved me out of the plane. But here I was, in free fall. Could we forcibly administer HIV medications? "I'd like to explain where I'm coming from. What we know about your condition and what we still need to figure out.

"Wasting your breath, Em."

But the skydiving analogy didn't seem apt. In truth, I was far from a model patient—I routinely ignored the medical advice to wear sunscreen despite my family's history of melanoma—but why?

"Sometimes," I said, considering what to say next. "Sometimes we do things . . ."

And then I went for it. "I take HIV meds," I said quickly. "I'll take them with you." It felt good to say it. I said it again, this time slower and louder. "I'll take them with you."

"Oh, please."

"I will. I swear. I take them at home."

"Try again."

"I'm serious."

She squeezed my hand. "I'm blind, not naïve. Not—"

"I give you my word." Was this manipulative? Did it matter?

"You have HIV?" She felt for the remote control near her pillow.

"I might have HIV." I inched closer. I could feel my voice about to quiver, so I whispered. "I stuck myself the other day with a needle. The patient had AIDS. And . . ."

"And your fingers are crossed."

"Yeah."

She shook her head. "Ain't that the shit."

I cleared my throat. "Do me a favor. Just take one pill, one time."

I took both of her hands in mine like we were reciting May-December wedding vows. I had a vague sense that I was making progress. She was engaging more with me than I'd seen with other doctors, most of whom she immediately waved away. It wasn't much, but it was something.

I wondered what exactly she saw, staring at me. "Fine," she said. "One pill. One time."

"All right!" If Jim O'Connell could see me now! If there had been a wineglass I would've stepped on it. I suspected Dre was in denial about her illness, and I wanted her to break through that. I wanted her to become angry, I wanted her to pass through the stages of grief and accept that she had a very real, very treatable condition. I didn't care if she used marijuana; I didn't really care if she sold marijuana. I just wanted her to acknowledge what she was up against and realize she could win. Until that moment, I would remain frustrated. But here, I saw an opening.

"And if that goes okay," I said exuberantly, "we can do two. Two pills." She had at most a few months before it was too late. "And then, three."

"I said one pill. One time. Keep talking and I might change my mind."

I let go of her hands and stood up. "Wonderful. See you tomorrow morning."

Dre and I still needed to confront the spinal tap and to get her there, to get her to agree to the procedure, I would undoubtedly have to go deeper still, searching for other ways to connect with her.

Walking out of her room, for the first time, I felt like a real doctor. In the words of Baio, it was fucking cool.

25

"Great news," I said to Ashley the next morning. We had exactly thirty-seven minutes to discuss twelve patients. "I talked Dre into taking the HIV meds."

"I don't want to know what kind of freaky shit you had to do to get her to agree to that."

She broke into laughter and held up her palm. I touched mine to hers. "I almost got to second base." I was still feeling exuberant.

"You are sick." She smiled and grabbed her coffee. "So what cocktail are we giving her?"

"I suppose the all-in-one pill makes the most sense."

She smirked. "Atripla? Sorry. Wrong answer. Her strain is resistant. She'll need something else."

There was no other all-in-one HIV pill. "Shit."

"She'll need a combination of three or four pills," Ashley said. "Good news is we have some options."

"Said she'd only take one today. Maybe the one with the least side effects."

"Also not an option. You have to hit the virus simultaneously from a number of angles with several different pills. Giving her one pill could make her strain even more resistant."

"She said she'd only take one pill today."

"Well, it won't be one for HIV. That's a nonstarter."

I clenched my fists in frustration. My big breakthrough was already going south and I'd barely had time to celebrate it. Worse, I worried that this would set back my growing relationship with Dre. She might see the news as a betrayal, or think I was playing with her emotions and not just an idiot who didn't even check to see what kinds of pills she needed to take before trying to convince her to take them.

Just before rounds I made the long march to her room. I felt like a parent who'd canceled a trip to Disney World and was about to break the news to my kids.

"Bait and switch!" Dre howled when she heard the news. "Now it's four? No, thank you." She turned her back to me and pulled a sheet over her upper body.

"Why do you think I'm being such a pain in the ass?" I asked. I tried to maintain my composure, but exasperation was starting to peek through. She didn't move. We were back at square one. "Talk to me."

"You have no idea, Em."

She was right, I didn't. I moved across the room and reentered her field of vision. My eyes were once again drawn to the innumerable lumps on her tiny face. I pulled a chair close to her bed and took a seat and began to plead my case. Did I have a case? Or should I just apologize for failing to understand the complexity of her disease? I explained how the medication worked, and why taking multiple pills was the only way to tackle her strain of the virus. But Dre was in no mood to listen. After twenty minutes of Beckettian back-and-forth, I threw in the towel and agreed to take one of my HIV pills—raltegravir—in return for her ingestion of a magnesium supplement. It was a paltry victory; we really only worried about magnesium supplementation in patients with cardiac problems. Dre had a number of issues, but heart disease wasn't one of them.

"Thank you," I said as my pager went off. "Progress." The spinal tap discussion would have to wait.

YOUR PRESENCE IS REQUESTED IN THE CCU ASAP

"Let's go for two pills tomorrow," I said, closing the door before she had a chance to answer.

The page made me nervous—everything in the hospital was done ASAP—which made someone writing it out in a text page seem suspicious. The CCU was my old stomping grounds, where I had first met Baio, first met Ariel and Meghan and Lalitha, and where I had first encountered Carl Gladstone. I mostly considered the Gladstone chapter behind me; I had learned from a colleague that he had been transferred to a rehab facility and was expected to make a full recovery. I hustled down four flights of stairs into the CCU, reflexively whispering "ABC, ABC" until I was intercepted by Mark, a cointern.

"Matisyahu!" he said, standing in the center of the unit with his hands on his hips. He had closely cropped, fire engine red hair and wore wire-rimmed glasses.

"Still trying to make that happen?" I asked.

"Got my page?" he asked. Mark, my puckish colleague, was informally known as the social chair of our intern class, always arranging happy hours and beer pong tournaments.

"Yeah," I said, holding up the pager. "What's up?"

He ran a finger across his upper lip. "Mustache race! You in?"

I was still thinking about Dre. The bait and switch, as she'd put it, had definitely been a step back for us. Seeing Jim O'Connell work his magic had not quite left me prepared for the complicated, delicate trust building that it must have taken him to reach his most difficult patients. I remembered Sheryl, and the six years it took Jim just to get her to agree to one therapy session. I could see now how slow the process would be with Dre. It might take me weeks or even months to get to her, time she barely had. I should have been back with her right then instead of down in the CCU talking about a goofy contest. Would Dre or any of the other patients care if the interns suddenly sprouted mustaches? The question prompted thoughts of Axel and his nuggets of doctorly wisdom—don't wear a bow tie, don't buy a motorcycle—and I imagined him ripping into me for the mustache.

Then the image of Dre's off-white eyeballs came to mind; they were like two igloos, flipped on their sides. Her words stung me, and I suddenly wanted a distraction. Luckily, there was one right in front of me. I put my hands on my hips, mimicking Mark. "I believe I am. I'm in."

I looked around the unit—it was strange to be back—and felt relief knowing that I wasn't responsible for any of the patients. This was a social visit. "I really can't wait," I said, feigning a bit of enthusiasm in the name of professional camaraderie. It occurred to me that the next time I'd be working in the unit, it would be as a second-year resident, teaching an unseasoned intern how to be a doctor.

"Nice! Gloria is going to judge. Be great for morale."

Gloria was the residency program's senior administrator—an ageless, zaftig Latina who never missed a chance to socialize.

"I should warn you," I said, "mine comes in red."

"Amazing!"

Mark seemed perfectly at home in the unit, somehow insulated from the weight of his work. Like Baio and Moranis, he genuinely seemed to enjoy practicing medicine. I wondered what his secret was. I had noticed how many interns, myself included, appeared at times to be faking it. Putting on a smile when we were delirious with exhaustion or enthusiastically offering to transport a patient or draw blood when in reality, we just wanted to go home and eat dinner. The gilded personas were omnipresent, but Mark was different—he didn't seem like the kind of guy who would dwell on mistakes or on success. He would probably try his best with Dre and then move on.

"Hey, that's your guy over there, right?" Levity evaporated as Mark pointed to the bed formerly inhabited by Professor Gladstone. A crowd of doctors and nurses hovered in front of the room. "Didn't I see you talking to him the other day?"

I stood on the balls of my feet and saw Benny, who looked like he was on a roller coaster—his teeth were clenched as he tightly gripped the bed's guardrails. "Oh, shit," I said softly, "shit shit." He was gasping for air when an anesthesiologist stepped in and obscured my view.

"He flashed," Mark said. "Not sure what tipped him over. Probably have to intubate." *Flashing* meant his lungs were suddenly over-whelmed with fluid, like a flash flood. It happens when the heart fails to pump sufficiently; blood backs up into the lungs and creates a sensation of drowning. A common culprit, particularly for a guy like Benny who was waiting for a new heart, was dietary indiscretion. I thought of the Snickers bar. "Jesus."

I wanted to run over to him, but the room was full. Someone was about to attach Benny to a ventilator. I clutched my chest, anticipating the phantom pain of a large tube sliding down my own throat. But I felt nothing. I just stood there, stunned at what I was seeing. Benny was drowning in front of my eyes, drowning in his own bodily fluids. How could I be so powerless to help him? Or to help Dre, for that matter? A resident tilted Benny's head back, and the large plastic tube was snaked down his throat. A moment later, a machine was breathing for him. A narcotic was quickly plunged into his IV to ensure he was sufficiently sedated.

"Hope he makes it," Mark said.

He sounded like any doctor with a healthy emotional investment in his patients' outcomes. I wasn't that doctor. I didn't know what I'd do if Benny didn't make it. "Fuck."

Mark glanced at his pager as we stretched to get a better view of Benny. Mark lightly punched my left arm. "Looking forward to the epic 'stache. Now back to work."

And with that he strolled into Gladstone's old room and calmly ordered a series of medications designed to remove the fluid from Benny's lungs as I looked on, frozen in space. The smiling man who could ride a stationary bike for an hour couldn't safely eat a Snickers bar without causing a flash flood in his lungs. On tiptoes, I stared blankly at the ventilator until my pager went off: YO, WHERE ARE YOU?—ASH

I silenced the pager, pulled out my scut list, and headed back to the HIV floor. In the hallway, I ran into Baio, who was staring down a vending machine. I sidled up next to him and looked at the row of Snickers bars. We hadn't had a substantive conversation since our time in the CCU together. I wondered if he knew about my mishap on the HIV floor.

"I heard," he said, carefully inserting a crumpled dollar bill. "Fuckin' sucks, man."

Of course he knew. "Word travels fast."

He stared intently at the machine as it spat out his dollar again and again. I wanted to take the bill and insert it myself—to say something clever and walk away. The teacher becomes the student or something.

"You'll get through it," he said. "You will."

"Yeah," I said. "You wouldn't believe all the pills." I was due to take another in half an hour.

"Hey, at least the guy didn't have hep C."

"Funny you mention that."

"No!" he said, running his hands through his hair.

"I went back and looked. HIV and hep C. Daily double."

I wondered what he saw when he looked at me. Did he ever wonder what I was doing in the hospital? How I was progressing as a physician? Did he ever think about our time together in the CCU?

"You'll be okay," he said.

"Hope so."

"No doubt."

The machine accepted his dollar. "Is that a thing," I asked, "just tell everyone they're going to be okay?"

"Nah."

"Really?"

He smiled and patted me on the back. "Yeah, it's a thing."

26

The sky was slate gray the next morning as I stepped out of my Upper West Side apartment building and headed to the subway, reformulating my case to Dre. It had been all I could think about overnight, as I read and reread the various notes I'd made to myself throughout the previous day. When I had gotten home from work, Heather could tell I was in need of a distraction and had taken me out to a BYOB Indian restaurant to get my mind off things. But I found myself unable to talk with her about anything other than the hospital—my patients, my pills—and I doubled over after I tried to take my first sip of beer.

I wasn't much of a conversationalist with her these days; I picked at my tikka masala as I stared off into space, trying in vain to divorce work life from my private life. But I was consumed by thoughts of Dre and Benny and of my own medical condition. Heather offered reassurance on a daily (and sometimes hourly) basis, but it was of little use. We both knew statistics were on my side, but what if I was the outlier? Shortly after boxing up the leftovers, I crawled into bed and drifted off to sleep, returning to Dre and the lumps on her face. She ultimately needed to be on nine different medications, which I hoped to achieve, one by one, as soon as possible.

It had been a fitful night of sleep—I'd scarfed down the leftover Indian food at 3:00 A.M. and spent the next hour checking my email— but as I strolled toward the uptown subway station, just as the morning sun was rising above the East River, I realized that Ashley was right. Under her gruff exterior, Dre did kinda like me. It wasn't quite like the relationships Jim O'Connell had with his patients, but it was something. It might give me enough of a toehold to get past the bait and switch. As I hopped on the 1 train toward Washington Heights, the idea of a career spent using unconventional methods to work with only the most difficult cases took hold of me.

Oh, McCarthy's the guy who touches faces. Like an even weirder Patch Adams, he's not for everyone, but there's a method to his—

A lavatorial whiff of the 168th Street subway stop—sulfur and saliva today—cued me that it was time to stop daydreaming. As I stepped into the Tuberculator, my thoughts returned to the silver screen and my favorite movie, *Groundhog Day,* where Bill Murray relives the same day again and again. Life at Columbia, which often took on a cinematic quality, was the antithesis of that film. I liked to think that was a good thing. My experiences outside of work, by contrast, were relatively unremarkable. When Heather and I could eat, we ate; when we could sleep, we slept. And if the mood struck us, we devoured episodes of *Lost.* But the needle stick had upended all of that. Now I routinely found myself at home, nodding through dinner or staring at a wall, trying to regain the physical and emotional energy to handle the rigors of my job, while contemplating an uncertain future and uncomfortable possibilities.

The news wasn't all bad. Benny had been stabilized and was expected to come off the ventilator in the next twenty-four hours, after the fluid was removed from his lungs, and Ashley had commended me in front of Dr. Chanel for convincing Dre to take the magnesium supplement. They were small victories, but they felt like something I could build on.

"Two pills," I said to myself over and over as I approached the hospital. "I know you can do it, Dre."

I exited the elevator and made a beeline for Dre's room. I knocked on the door and called her name, but there was no response. "It's Em," I said loudly as I opened the door. The room was empty. "Dre?" I wrinkled my brow and wondered where she could be. Patients often left the floor for imaging studies, but I hadn't scheduled anything for her. As I stared at her empty bed, an elderly white woman was wheeled into the room by a nurse.

"Where's Dre?" I asked.

The nurse shook his head. "Who?"

"The woman who was in this room yesterday." Patients were occasionally shuffled around based on the male-female ratio of beds and at times were clustered in rooms based on their histories of communicable diseases. "Tiny black woman," I said, holding my hand up to my hip.

"Oh," he said, helping the woman into bed. "Gone."

"Yeah. Where?" I didn't have much time before rounds, and nothing was quick with Dre.

"She's gone, man."

"What?"

"Left in the middle of the night."

"What? How?"

"Grabbed her stuff and left."

"She's blind. She can't just leave."

"Just grabbed her stuff in the middle of the night and left."

I shook my head. "That's impossible."

"Security tried to stop her, but she's gone."

My arms went limp; I felt like I'd been kicked in the stomach. I hadn't been aware until just that moment how emotionally sucked into Dre's life I had become. The face touching, the playful nicknames, the agreement to take one pill. We were connecting. At least I had thought we were. Now I wondered if I'd imagined the whole thing. What if that was just how she was with everyone? I had assumed I was special when I wasn't, and it hurt.

And I had told her that I might have HIV. That had seemed fine in the moment, when we were making progress, but now I felt vulnerable and uneasy about it, not to mention guilty. In the cold light of her absence, that level of sharing seemed manipulative. She was a poor homeless woman who suffered terribly from the disease. I was a doctor who wasn't even sure he had it. It was hardly the equivalency I had presented to her. Maybe she saw through it. Maybe she hated me for bringing it up and using it to play on her sympathy.

It mattered all the more because Dre was my responsibility. Lalitha may have checked her in overnight, but technically Chanel and I were her doctors. I felt like I had failed her. She was headed out into the world without HIV meds, and she would be dead in a few months because I couldn't get through to her. This sort of thing never happened to Jim O'Connell.

My body sagged as I exited the room and walked down the hall. I wanted to talk with someone. I wanted to go to Wendy's and have another Frosty with Ariel. I couldn't move on, but I had to. There were more patients to see, more notes to write. I closed my eyes tightly as four words began bouncing around my head: *Why did she go?*

PART III

27

"I don't want to screw you."

Meghan's words slapped me across the face at 10:00 P.M., several weeks after Dre had gone AWOL. Our pod had moved from the infectious diseases service to the general medicine floor, and tonight it was my turn to work the thirty-hour shift. The floor housed patients with rather mundane illnesses—blood clots, alcohol withdrawal, bellyaches—as well as patients with mysterious illnesses who couldn't be assigned to a specialized floor because no one could figure out what was wrong with them. It was unclear why Meghan was still bouncing around the nurses' station. She should have gone home hours ago. And what the hell was she talking about?

"I'm sorry?" I mumbled, stoop-shouldered and pondering a tray of leftover donuts as she blew past me. I waved my hand to get her attention, but her focus was elsewhere. In search of a nurse, Meghan held up a finger in my direction and mouthed, "One sec."

I sat down at a computer and began reviewing a brain MRI. Lalitha and Ariel had handed me their scut lists and signed over their pagers hours ago and in doing so transferred a potential maelstrom of unfinished business. The idea was to keep the to-do list as short as possible because the evening's transition of care was inherently fraught with complications. I'd never met their patients and had my own new admissions to distract me through the sleepless night, so situationally I was much more likely to misinterpret a symptom or concern. But these handoffs were an inevitable and increasingly prevalent part of medicine. I'd heard some hospitals even taught the art of the transition during orientation. They may have done it at Columbia, but if so I'd missed it.

"Sorry, I didn't want to screw you." Meghan pulled up a chair ten minutes later. "I got fucked," she said, pointing at her scut list, "last time I was on call. Totally destroyed." She pulled out a scrunchie from the back pocket of her scrubs and slipped it around her blond hair.

"Oh?" I glanced with some relief at the sparse list she was about to hand me.

"Today's been a nightmare."

"What happened?"

She tilted her head toward the step-down unit—an enclosed room for patients who were seriously ill but just missed the cut for an ICU. "Drug mule," she said.

"Like an actual drug mule?" I asked, looking over at the unit. "*Maria Full of Grace* drug mule?"

"Nineteen-year-old swallowed sixteen bags of heroin in the Dominican and hopped on a flight to JFK."

"Holy shit." It was never Groundhog Day at Columbia.

"Then jumped in a cab and came straight to our emergency room and confessed. DR to the ER."

"Whoa."

"She's just been pooping them out one at a time, handcuffed to the hospital bed. Cop sitting right next to her."

"And this has to be done in step-down?"

"If one of those bags rips she's dead."

"Yikes."

She handed me her scut list. "Only thing I need you to do tonight is a poop check."

"Poop check?"

"Make sure she keeps crapping out those heroin bags. Constipation could kill her. If she stops pooping, get a CAT scan. And if there's an obstruction, call surgery."

"I believe I can handle that."

Like most of us, Meghan had a hard time letting go. Every day felt like an unfinished, complicated work in progress with a jumble of loose ends, and there was always a reason to stay another hour in the hospital. Doctors were fond of saying that the later you stay, the later you stay. This meant that friendships and romantic relationships took a backseat and in many cases, began to fade. I had a hard time imagining what I would talk about with my college buddies who lived in Manhattan and worked in finance.

"I must've sifted through a hundred thousand dollars' worth of her shit today," Meghan said. "Unbelievable."

I tried to imagine the life circumstances that would lead a teenager to swallow expensive narcotics and hop on an airplane. As I scribbled down *poop check,* our pagers blared simultaneously.

FREE MUSTACHE RIDES IN THE CCU!

Meghan shook her head. "You guys are having way too much fun with this."

The page reminded me of Benny. I had continued to check in on him after the breathing tube had been removed from his throat. They weren't long visits, just enough to peek in and confirm he was improving. Once he regained the ability to speak, we talked football and watched the Yankees. It was remarkable how close he could get to dying and how little beaten down or fazed by the experience he seemed a few weeks later. I wished I had his resilience.

Sometimes I tried to convince myself that his mild progress mirrored my own. As I gradually became more capable, more confident, more efficient, his heart would become stronger and his lungs drier. But deep down, I knew that wasn't fair. We were two random people thrown together, and our challenges were wildly unrelated. My success or failure as a doctor had nothing to do with his quest to get a heart. But I liked telling myself it did. I liked thinking that when I had finally mastered all of the skills it took to be a doctor, Benny would finally get his transplant.

Meghan stood up and grabbed her purse.

"CCU?" I asked with a smile.

"Bed," she said. "Good luck tonight."

At 2:00 A.M., after every task but one had been scratched off the scut list, I grabbed a pair of disposable gloves and headed to the step-down unit to perform the poop check. When I entered the dimly lit room, I could vaguely make out the face of a teenage Hispanic woman—a girl, really—handcuffed to a bed, quietly sobbing. Next to her was a police officer seated in an orange plastic chair with the *New York Post* in his lap. The officer put down the paper and waved me in.

"Dr. McCarthy," I said, approaching them. "Covering for the day team."

A muted television in the corner of the dark room illuminated their faces. The patient was short and thin with long black hair, and I could see tears trickling down her cheeks. Thin red bruises spanned the circumference of each wrist, and the top of her light blue hospital gown was a damp reservoir of tears. Between the cop and her distraught condition, I immediately felt uncomfortable. What was I participating in? What would happen to this woman after she finally pooped out all the bags? Was it a straight trip with the cop from here to jail, and then back to whatever awful situation had compelled her to do this in the first place? I slipped on the gloves and placed a hand on her shoulder.

"Ayúdame," she said as I stood over her. *Help me.*

I placed the stethoscope into my ears and looked at the cop. "Just here to get her through the night." He nodded, and I dropped the instrument onto the woman's thin abdomen. Her soft belly gently swayed up and down as I tried to listen for bowel sounds, but all I could hear were muffled sobs. My neck stiffened in response to her outpouring of emotion. Dre flashed in my mind.

"Ayúdame," she said again.

I looked at her midsection and imagined the tiny bags of narcotics lying just beneath the surface, swimming through her intestines. I gently pressed the tips of my fingers into her belly, trying to elicit a subtle sign of pain or tenderness, something that might indicate that a bag had burst, but there was nothing. I removed the stethoscope and examined her face, wondering again what life circumstances had brought this woman to this moment.

But just as quickly as I began to wonder, I felt my mind closing, and a kind of self-protective numbness set in. There was certainly a part of me that wanted to know more about her—her life, her family, why she swallowed drugs for money—but even the thought of reaching out produced a small burst of shame, and brought back the anger I'd felt at seeing Dre's empty bed. Sure, I still wanted to be like Jim O'Connell, but the reality of connecting with patients was far more difficult than I'd ever imagined. It was messy, and had the potential to make me messy, too, something I desperately wanted to avoid. Emotionally investing in patients was important, but it was going to take a backseat to all of the other tasks I had on my scut list.

I tapped her handcuffed wrist. *"Lo siento,"* I said. *I'm sorry.*

Ignoring this woman's tears made me feel like a machine. Was this what the Badass felt like when he saw patients? I looked at the officer. "I need to sift through her feces."

He pointed to a plastic blue bin about the size of a top hat in the corner of the room that was filled with a frothy brown liquid. I stepped away from the woman, brought the bin over to a sink, and dipped my gloved index finger into it, fishing around for a plastic bag. I breathed through my mouth to avoid the odor and was careful not to splash any of the refuse onto the floor.

"No drugs," I said a moment later. *"Nada."* I looked back at the woman and removed my gloves. Her large dark eyes continued to emit a stream of tears. The officer shrugged and returned to the newspaper.

"Ayúdame," she said once more.

I shook my head. "I'll be back in a few hours," I said flatly, "to do this again." Then I walked out of the room and shut the door.

I was headed, as had become all too common, to the bathroom for another urgent death match with my bowels. Several weeks into taking the HIV pills, I now had a clear understanding of why patients sometimes refused them. Ritonavir, the pill that looked like an astronaut meal, seemed to get stuck in my throat every time I tried to swallow it, and the first wave of side effects included an ever-present feeling of fullness that shrank my appetite to subdiet levels. Then I started experiencing gnawing pains and cramps that would manifest unpredictably in various parts of my belly. Pain came during meals or not, and before long I was having phantom stomach pains that began the moment I put the pill in my mouth.

What being a doctor gave me in perspective it took away through overeducation. I knew what tenofovir could do to my kidneys, and the damage ritonavir might wreak on my liver, and soon these organs started hurting, too, even though tests showed no problems. Walking around the hospital feeling light-headed, I wondered if it was kidney dehydration or just a mindfuck. Clearly not phantom was the diarrhea. I had taken up Dr. Chanel on her offer of Zofran for nausea, further increasing my pill burden.

As I exited the bathroom once again, feeling shaken and worse for the wear, I tried to think about the crying woman in step-down, but I didn't have it in me. Between getting burned by Dre and feeling like a shell of myself thanks to the pills, I had very little bandwidth to connect with my patients beyond trying to keep them alive. Every time I thought of my patient's pain, I thought of my pain, and of the medications that were causing it. Every time I imagined taking the pills for the rest of my life, I wanted to scream.

———

In the midst of my third and final poop check, a few minutes before 7:00 A.M., my pager went off. The message was just a phone number, and a moment later, I found myself on the phone with an oncologist named Dr. Phillips. One of his patients—a middle-aged Cuban woman with multiple myeloma—had been hospitalized with pneumonia and I was taking care of her on the general medicine service. I had never met Dr. Phillips, but he left notes in the woman's chart, explaining what he wanted me to do for her on a given day.

"I need you to come to my office," he said, as I held the phone in one hand and my soiled gloves in another. "As soon as possible."

I was at the tail end of a thirty-hour shift and my brain was starting to shut down; soon my vision would be blurry and my judgment would be grossly impaired. I didn't want to meet him. "Is it something we can talk about over the phone?" I asked. "It's just that I'm post-call and we've got rounds that go till noon."

"I will see you in my office as soon as rounds are over."

What could this be about? I wondered. What couldn't be said over the phone? Or via email? Whatever it was, it didn't sound good, and I wasn't remotely in the mood for bad news.

Just after noon, I staggered into Dr. Phillips's wood-paneled office. There was an orchid on his desk and the usual column of diplomas on the wall. He had white hair and a long, broad nose. He offered me a seat in a large brown leather chair as he remained standing behind his desk.

"Dr. McCarthy," he said, "thank you for meeting me face-to-face."

"Of course. It's nice to finally meet you in pers——."

"You're taking care of Ms. Barroso," he said, loudly clasping his hands together. "I've known her a long time. A very long time."

"Yes." I quickly scanned my brain for the latest details of her case. "Seems to be doing well. Hopefully discharged in a few days."

"Tell me, Dr. McCarthy, what happens to vital signs when a patient is in pain?"

This was what couldn't be asked over the phone? My eyes were heavy and my stomach ached; I was due for another round of HIV pills. Why was he doing this to me? "Heart rate and blood pressure increase," I said. "Although I'm sure there are exceptions."

He nodded. "Now tell me, do her relatively unremarkable vital signs tell you anything about whether Ms. Barroso is in pain?"

It felt like a trick question. I flashed back on my conversation with Sothscott over Gladstone. My neck started to tingle. "Not necessarily."

He took a seat and frowned. "Dr. McCarthy, Ms. Barroso has been in agony for several days. She's suffering." He shook his head and locked eyes with me. "And it's because of you."

I was suddenly very awake; I felt every muscle in my body clench. "What?"

"I asked you to come to my office because I need an explanation. I need to hear from you why this is happening."

I shook my head and sat up in my chair as words leapt out of my mouth. "Every day I ask her, *Tienes dolor?* Do you have pain? And she says no. Every single day. This is the first I'm hearing that she's in pain."

He put his elbows on his desk and wrinkled his brow. "Do you use a translator?"

"No, I don't. I ask her in Spanish if she's in pain and she says no." He shook his head.

"I ask her every day," I added. I could tell my words were coming out too quickly, that I sounded defensive. I tried to slow down, but I couldn't. "The nurses ask her every shift. If she said yes, they'd page me. But they haven't paged me."

He shook his head. "She's suffering."

Were we talking about the same patient? "I must be missing something."

"Indeed."

This wasn't making sense. "I'm running all over the hospital and no one has ever paged me to—"

"Has it ever occurred to you that you're not using the right words? That you're not asking the right questions?"

I paused. "Honestly, no."

"If you bothered to get a translator, you might understand that she's in agony."

Bothered? Was he claiming I'd been negligent? "I feel terrible about this, but I'm not sure what to say."

"Apologize. And use a translator."

I stared down at my shoes, trying to make sense of this conversation. I was deliriously sleep-deprived, but this had nothing to do with that. "I'm deeply sorry, but it has never been communicated to anyone that she's suffering. And I can't have a translator just following me around."

He clenched his teeth. "It was communicated to me. And there are phone translators in every room." He scribbled down a phone number on an index card and handed it to me. "Use it."

I looked at the numbers and tried to wrap my head around what was happening. I took a deep breath. "Okay."

He closed his eyes and sighed. "That's it. That's all I have to say. I'll give you one more chance to get this right."

Then what? I was too scared to ask.

28

Two days later I found myself sitting cross-legged in a group circle in Palisades, New York, at the intern retreat, where for twenty-four hours we were given a much-needed respite from hospital life. It was a crisp afternoon at the IBM Executive Conference Center, a corporate refuge with tennis courts, saunas, and walking trails. Geese walked by as eight of us—one attending physician and seven interns—sat next to a small pond. The retreat was an opportunity to clear our heads— *mental hygiene* was the phrase of the day—but I couldn't stop reliving the past forty-eight hours. The delirious interaction in Dr. Phillips's office felt like a bad dream. I didn't think I was wrong, but I hated to think a patient might be suffering because of me. And getting dressed down by Phillips about my competence in the wake of the needlestick and Dre's departure made me ashamed and nervous.

"It's a heck of a year," the attending said. "This is a chance to just talk, off the record, about how things are going. No judgment."

She was tall and thin with sandy-blond hair and a mole on her left cheek and had been in our position a half dozen years earlier. She turned to her right and nodded. "You first."

The physician to her right, a thin, mustachioed Indian man hoping to become a cardiologist, held up his palms and said "Great," then turned to his right.

"Excellent" came next.

"Fantastic. Every day I show up to work and witness a miracle."

I rolled my eyes. No chinks in the armor of enthusiasm.

"Really wonderful."

These were not the words coming to my mind. I could hear Baio's voice whispering, *Everyone breaks.*

"Incredible."

Twenty-four hours earlier, I'd gone down to the CCU to visit Benny, who now appeared gaunt and frail. Buds of gray hair sprang up from his normally bald scalp, and he spoke in one- and two-word sentences. The past few weeks had been hell for him, and the intubation process had reminded him just how close he was to death. It had been a mistake to conflate his physical health with my mental health. Life inside the hospital was like life outside the hospital—unpredictable and unfair. The intern to my left touched my shoulder—my turn.

"Well, it's been a challenge," I said, thinking of Gladstone and Dre and Dr. Phillips and my most recent bout of radioactive diarrhea. "I've learned a lot, but I wouldn't say it's been great." I saw a mix of nods and blank faces; I felt for one of the pills in my pocket and rubbed it against my thigh. I was due for an HIV test in just under two weeks. It loomed on the horizon like Judgment Day.

The attending leaned in. "Would you like to talk more about that?"

I thought about all the shit that I'd been through. Intern year had worn me down—I could feel myself getting burned out—and I didn't know how to stop it. I looked around the circle at the vaguely familiar faces and realized I had spent very little time with the interns outside of my pod. Meghan, Lalitha, Ariel, and I had grown a bit closer as the year had worn on—taking trips to Wendy's whenever we could steal away a few moments from the hospital. We talked about families and past lives—Lalitha and I discovered that we had been in the same organic chemistry class as undergraduates—but mostly we just vented. We talked about the occasional ups but mostly the downs: the tongue-lashings and errors and sleepless nights. It was difficult for each of us, but in different ways. We promised to keep the frustrations within our close-knit group of four, remembering that no one wants to hear from a whiny doctor.

"This is a safe space," the attending said, prompting me to elaborate.

"Maybe later," I muttered. I didn't feel like sharing with this group of relative strangers. The old intern code of protection kicked in: mistakes are signs of weakness, and these people didn't really know me. Vulnerability wasn't the first impression I wanted to make.

It struck me how different this was from medical school, where I was friendly with just about everyone. We had classes in the morning, studied in the afternoon, and congregated in dorm rooms or apartments at night to socialize or study more. But in Manhattan, everyone lived separate, anonymous, exhausted lives.

"Certainly," the attending replied and moved on to the woman next to me.

"Really rewarding," she said.

"Okay, great," our leader said. "So . . . I want this to be an opportunity to just talk. I have a few questions I'll throw out to the group."

A goose approached the circle, and someone threw a pebble at it.

"Has anyone seen something in the hospital that traumatized them?"

Silence followed by muffled laughter. "Where would I begin?" said another Indian physician, this one with a scruffy beard.

"Yes," said a brunette. "Almost every day."

Something had changed. You could see in the uncomfortable shifting around the circle that the question had shaken something loose. I wondered if each of my cointerns had an adequate release valve, a way to blow off steam after an awful day.

Those of us who felt ground down had an uneasy relationship with the hospital's slogan: *Amazing Things Are Happening Here!* No doubt amazing things were happening every day, from breakthrough advances in treatment to saving lives that seemed lost; and part of the thrill was sharing in those successes. But some of us had no trouble in seeing the irony of the word *amazing*—the moments when getting spit on or physically threatened could leave you speechless. Many times, when sharing a particularly dispiriting story, an intern would turn the slogan on its head: "A patient barfed on me yesterday. *Twice*. Yep, amazing things are happening here." It had become a kind of mantra for interns, a coping mechanism for trying both to appreciate the great moments of doctoring and to contextualize the tough ones. I couldn't help but think the hospital PR office would have been aghast. But the more I thought about it, the more I considered it a brilliant tagline, a dead-on summation of our roller-coaster profession.

The leader smiled. "Would anyone like to elaborate?"

Eyes averted. More silence. "Okay, let's switch gears. Has anyone made what they would consider a medical error?"

No one spoke. It suddenly seemed like a great time to take in our surroundings. Were we having even remotely similar experiences? Were we all destined to break? Suddenly I heard myself speaking.

"I did," I said. I paused. I wasn't quite sure why I had opened my mouth. A moment earlier, I'd had no intention of speaking. But here I was, on the verge of opening up. And the funny thing was I felt better already, just having said "I did." It was the same feeling of relief I had experienced at Wendy's telling Ariel about the needle stick and when I'd opened up to Dre. I was not a doctor who could live with these things unspoken or unshared. Maybe it was as simple as that.

"Same," added the aspiring cardiologist.

"Me, too," said another.

The attending nodded at me to go on. It seemed like I had an embarrassment of riches when it came to mistakes—which one to choose? The needle stick was a medical error, certainly, but I didn't want to talk about that. Should I mention Dr. Phillips and his comment that he'd give me *one more chance to get this right*? I went with Gladstone. It felt the most resolved.

"In the CCU," I said quietly, "first week of work, I had a guy with anisocoria." Eyebrows rose, acknowledging the unusual condition.

"I thought it was medication-related. But it wasn't." I considered how much to divulge. "It was . . . it was actually something entirely different."

"I've done something like that," the brunette said quickly. All eyes focused on her. "I thought someone's cough was due to asthma," she said, blinking her bright blue eyes, "but I got a chest X-ray and it was actually a pleural effusion."

The attending smiled as the goose again approached our circle. "Matt, back to you. Did your patient have a bad outcome?"

I looked at the goose and softly said, "It's . . . complicated."

The attending rocked gently. "And, Matt," she asked, leaning toward me, "did you apologize?"

I attempted to swallow. I had not been expecting this follow-up question. "I did not." Heads hung; the brunette winced. "I wasn't sure how to do it," I said flatly. "Given the circumstances . . . I'm not sure it would've been appropriate. Someone else caught my error." In theory, there were a million reasons why I didn't apologize. But in reality there were none. I often thought I should've tracked down Gladstone's wife and explained that if not for Diego, I would've made a colossal oversight, and the ramifications of that oversight gave me nightmares for months. But what purpose would that have served? I regretted the entire episode, but airing my self-doubt with a family member seemed unwise.

I looked around the circle at each intern. It was different from intern report, where I'd been convinced I was observing gilded personas. Here I saw a mix of emotions—some faces smiling, pretending that life was *incredible!* or perhaps just relieved to have some time away from the hospital. But others appeared anguished, deep in thought about an incident that may have taken place in the hospital. We were all quietly reflecting on something. Soon the silence became uncomfortable; I ached for someone else to say something. Anything.

"I made a mistake once," the attending said. "Week before my wedding I had to put a chest tube in someone. The lung was filling up with fluid and the patient couldn't breathe. I made the incision and the tube slid right in. Easy peasy." She frowned and looked away from the group. "I sutured the person up, shot a chest X-ray, and realized I'd put the tube in the wrong lung." She bit her bottom lip and ran her hands through her hair. "I think about that chest tube every time I do a procedure. I was thinking about it a week later when I walked down the aisle."

29

Two days later and back in the hospital, I received a page from Dave, the chief resident who'd given the phlebotomy tutorial at intern report. I wasn't sure what it was about—the message only asked, YOU FREE?—and I quickly tried to recall if I'd said or done anything that would warrant a face-to-face discussion with an administrator.

My mind immediately leapt back to the Palisades retreat, which had ended up being a cathartic bonding experience with the other interns. The realization that I wasn't alone gave me the courage to really unburden myself; I'd ultimately described in detail what I'd gone through with Gladstone, with Peter and Denise, and with Dre, though I'd skipped the part about the needle stick. Over the course of the retreat, only a few people had refused to speak candidly. Many of my colleagues had opened up about what the daily traumas of medicine had done to their fragile psyches. The surprising part was how, despite all the vicissitudes of the recent months, I was not the most exhausted or damaged intern. During a group hike several of my fellow interns confided that they intended to leave the program before the end of the year. I felt better having heard their stories, but now I wondered if I'd said too much; if, despite the retreat having been a safe space, something had made its way back to Dave.

I tucked my pager back into its holster and headed toward the chief residents' office. There were four of them, and each chief resident had just completed the Columbia internal medicine residency program and was now spending the year arranging conferences, teaching medical students, and keeping tabs on the mental health of the residents. They were liaisons between residents and the hospital's administration, often serving as the bearers of bad news when a new regulation or oversight committee was foisted upon us. It was a great honor to be selected as a chief resident, and the position was frequently a pit stop for physicians applying for the ultracompetitive cardiology fellowships. (Diego had once been a chief resident.) I tried to imagine what the meeting was about as I hopped down three flights of stairs.

"What's up, guy?" Dave said as I entered the tiny, windowless room. On his desk were four pictures of an attractive woman doing yoga. "Take a seat."

"Hi, Dave." We had spoken a handful of times, mostly before and after educational conferences. He liked to put a hand on my shoulder when we talked, and he evoked the image of an assistant coach—someone who was there to advise and guide me, but lacking the gravitas of a senior physician. There was an off-the-record feel to our interactions; he knew what interns were going through because he'd been one just three years ago.

I sat down and crossed my legs. "How are you?" he asked eagerly.

I smiled. "You know . . . hanging in there."

He nodded vigorously and readjusted himself in his chair. "How do you feel?"

"I'm good."

I found myself staring at the yoga lady. Dave took off his glasses and we sat in silence. "I'm going to get right to the point," he said, clasping his hands together. "We're worried about you."

We locked eyes momentarily. "What?" I said.

"Five interns are leaving the program. That's unheard of."

It was true. I hadn't been aware of the deep discontent among my peers until the Palisades retreat. "Well," I said, with as much enthusiasm as I could muster, "I'm not going anywhere." I wondered why the departing doctors were all men. No answer sprang to mind.

Dave put his glasses back on. "I heard about the error. The thing with the pupils."

I flinched and looked away. It had taken place more than four months ago; why was he bringing it up now? Word must've trickled out from the retreat. "I thought that was confidential."

"I also know about the needle stick."

I felt a knot in my stomach; I wanted to know who else had spoken with him. I wondered if Dr. Phillips had told him about our conversation. Dave leaned back, pulled a handkerchief from his breast pocket, and blew his damp nostrils. I briefly closed my eyes and again felt the urge to disappear. "Look, people talk. What can I say?"

"You could say that stuff at the retreat isn't actually confidential."

His eyes scanned back and forth across my face. "Matt, this isn't meant to be an inquisition. I'm just checking in to see how you're doing."

That wasn't what it felt like. I was sick of the hot seat. "I'm . . . fine."

"You've been through a lot."

Ashley had once told me she didn't want to hear that I was struggling. The whole complex hierarchy made it impossible to figure out when it was safe to vent and when not. But I was running out of patience. "Okay, Dave, I'm not fine." I leaned back in my chair. "I'm not fine at all. Is that what you want to hear? I made mistakes, people are leaving the program, and . . ." The corner of his lip curled upward as he nodded. "And I might have AIDS."

"You don't have AIDS, Matt. But talking about this stuff is a good thing."

It was making me feel worse. I had to take the HIV pills for ten more days, and then it was time for the blood test. Then I would know if I'd contracted the virus. Why did Dave want to talk about this stuff now? As I thought about what to say next, my pager went off. Perfect. I was getting the hell out of there. "I need to respond to this," I said, without reading the message.

"Oh sure, sure," Dave said, pushing the phone in my direction.

"No, it's something on the floor," I said. "I have to go see a patient."

I extended my hand, and he smiled. "Good talk, Matt," he said. "Let's keep the lines of communication open."

I had no intention of doing so. I felt my nostrils flare; I wanted to hit something. "Sure thing."

I caught another glimpse of the downward-facing dog and walked to the stairwell.

30

A day later, while sitting in on an informal talk by Dr. Chanel on the emergence of multidrug-resistant tuberculosis, I received a page from my faculty adviser, Dr. Petrak. A former chief resident, Petrak was now the junior faculty member responsible for providing me with clinical wisdom and career guidance. He was, in theory, the guy who would help me decide if I wanted to become a rheumatologist or a cardiologist. I excused myself from rounds and walked down the hall to his office.

I knew that every few months, I was supposed to review my faculty evaluations with Petrak and figured he was paging me to do so. I expected the initial evaluations to be weak—the Badass had scolded me for not knowing how to properly read a chest X-ray—but I knew I had made substantial progress. Both Ashley and Dr. Chanel had complimented me on my bedside manner with angry patients, and on the general medicine service I'd convincingly demonstrated that I could perform a poop check.

As I entered the office, I took in the diplomas and certificates of achievement that hung just millimeters apart from one another on a crowded beige wall. Dr. Petrak—a forty-something Lithuanian with bushy black eyebrows—stood up and smiled. Small framed pictures of his family were scattered across his desk.

"Dr. McCarthy," he said, extending a hand. "Please . . . take a seat."

"Thank you."

The last time I had been in this office, a year earlier, Petrak was interviewing me for a spot in the residency program. Since then we had exchanged small waves and quick handshakes as we briskly passed each other in the hospital's lobby, but that had been the extent of our contact. "How are you?" he asked.

"Good," I said, removing my stethoscope from my neck and placing it in my coat pocket. "Very good."

"Good," he said as he sipped from a coffee mug. "Great."

We stared at each other for a moment before he cracked his knuckles. "The purpose of this meeting," he said, "is just to check in."

I took two quick breaths and found myself once again drawn to the eyebrows. Under the fluorescent lights, I noticed that they contained hints of gray, just like my own hair. I'd finished medical school with a thick brown mane, but I'd been discovering more thin gray hairs by the day. At first I wanted to blame the HIV medications, but I knew it wasn't that. It must be the overwhelming workload; I had aged several years in several months.

"So . . ." Petrak said as he pointed an index finger at me, "how are you?"

These conversations all seemed to be the same way. "Like I said, I'm good." I held up a computer printout of my patient's vital signs. "You know, staying busy."

"Good, good." The eyebrows bounced on his forehead; you could probably braid those fucking things. "So here's the deal," he said. "I talked to Dave and a few other people."

"Okay."

"And I hear you've been through a lot."

I leaned back in my chair. "Huh."

"What can I say?" he said, shrugging his shoulders. "People talk."

"I'm aware."

"People are worried about you. Interns are dropping out and we need to identify those who might—"

"I'm okay."

"People are worried you are . . . how do I say . . . decompensating."

"Decompensating?"

"Yes."

It was a word I had never used before coming to Columbia, but now I heard it tossed around all the time. *To decompensate* meant *to unravel.* We used the term to describe clinical phenomena—Benny's failing heart was in the process of decompensating—and to describe emotional turmoil. A frazzled intern who appeared to be on the verge of snapping, or who was seen yelling at a nurse or a patient, was said to be decompensating. It was a word that at some point could be applied to every intern. I might have used it to describe myself earlier in the year, but not now. Petrak took another sip, and I folded my arms. "I don't know what to say."

"You don't have to say anything, Matt. But for your own sake, I want you to know that you're now operating under a microscope. People are watching you. We don't want to lose any more interns."

"Okay."

"And they may begin to question your clinical decision making."

My thoughts flashed to Dr. Phillips. Had he said something to Petrak? Was that what this was about? I carefully considered my words. "Are people questioning my decisions?" I asked.

"No."

"Well, that's good." I took another deep breath. Were these kinds of threats or warnings common?

"Not yet."

"Oh."

Operating under a microscope? Was increased observation supposed to prevent me from decompensating or precipitate my decompensation? I ran my hands through my hair, and the specter of Carl Gladstone in a rehabilitation facility flashed across my mind. In its place appeared a vision of Magic Johnson giving me a high five in a public service announcement for HIV. Soon Banderas was going to draw my blood and call me with the results. I tried to imagine him saying, *I have some bad news.*

"Look, Matt," Petrak said after a long pause, "I'm only telling you this for your own benefit."

The meeting concluded a moment later. I stepped out of his office and apparently into the crosshairs of the microscope. "You have got to be fucking kidding me," I said softly as I approached a vending machine next to the hospital's elevator. I smacked the machine's Plexiglas with the palm of my hand. "Fuck!" An Orthodox Jewish couple walked by, and I sheepishly took off my white coat and pager. I couldn't remember the last time I'd hit anything in anger. "Fuck!" I said and again slammed the machine.

I had never felt lower. The entire chain of command appeared worried that I might either leave or accidentally kill a patient if I stayed. No one seemed angry; in fact the overriding attitude from both Dave and Petrak was concern. But it didn't make me feel any better. I was living day to day in constant pain, creeping closer to a verdict on my future health, and every time I thought about it, I thought about what an awful stupid fucking mistake I'd made to be in this position. Over the months I had become better at so many aspects of being a doctor, but it wasn't enough. Not enough for me, not enough for Dre, not for Phillips and his patient, and apparently not for the people who were supposed to be looking out for me.

If I had blown off any steam at intern retreat, it had just come back with reinforcements. As I wound up for a third shot at the vending machine, the overhead intercom went off.

ARREST STAT, SEVEN HUDSON NORTH! ARREST STAT, SEVEN HUDSON NORTH!

I grabbed my coat and was off, sprinting down two flights of stairs. *ABC, ABC...*

I bounded past Moranis—he was giving a tour of the hospital to a group of medical school applicants—and was the third person to arrive at the bedside of a twenty-one-year-old African-American woman who had been found unresponsive by her nurse. I thought of Baio's hypotheticals in the cardiac care unit as the arrest resident arrived a moment later. She quickly gave orders—chest compressions, defibrillator, epinephrine—before turning to me and saying, "Central access."

Shit. My job was to insert a large-bore IV into the young woman's groin, a procedure I'd done just once before. Learning medicine was about being thrown into the fire, learning on the fly, but since I'd left the CCU, I'd been dealing with different types of fires. My patients on the infectious diseases service were not critically ill, in the strictest sense of the term, and as a result, they hadn't needed the critical care that I'd learned in the CCU. So I felt uncomfortable inserting this enormous IV, but I knew I had to do it. I imagined the lens of a giant microscope hovering above me.

I reached for the central line kit and took a deep breath. I did not want to do this procedure. I didn't want to fuck up and I didn't want administrators to talk about me. But there was no time for my existential crisis. The room became more and more crowded as I swabbed the young woman's groin with iodine. I could feel blood coursing through her femoral artery with each chest compression. An anesthesiologist quickly snaked a breathing tube into her trachea.

"No pulse for four minutes," the arrest resident said to the group. "Let's go."

I uncapped the large needle and moved it toward the woman's right hip. Her lifeless body bounded like a rag doll's as the team performed CPR. I told myself to breathe. I briefly closed my eyes and thought of the anatomy. Ashley taught me to remember the anatomical location of the vessels in the groin with the mnemonic NAVEL. Starting from the hip and moving inward, the order is:

N—femoral nerve
A—femoral artery

V—femoral vein
E—empty space
L—lymphatics

The IV has to be inserted in the femoral vein; striking the artery or nerve would be devastating. The only vessel you can feel is the artery. Once it's identified, the needle is inserted medially, striking the vein. If deep purple blood fills the syringe, you've hit your target; bright red blood means you've landed squarely in the artery. I imagined Dave, Dr. Phillips, and Petrak in the corner of the room, whispering about what I might do wrong.

I took a deep breath and shoved the needle, which was attached to a large syringe, into the woman's leg. Pulling back on the syringe, I slowly advanced the needle, waiting to see it fill with blood. There was nothing.

I pulled back and inserted the needle again as the young body bounced. It was critical to get the IV into the vein as quickly as possible so that the powerful, potentially lifesaving medications could be rapidly administered. My heart was racing, my breathing ragged. Sweat pooled under my arms. Several physicians looked on as I fished around inside her pelvis, wondering if I was in the E of NAVEL. The hole in her punctured skin became a bit larger every time I readjusted the needle.

"Eight minutes without a pulse," the arrest resident announced. "And does anyone know if she's pregnant? Matt, how are we doing on access?"

Pregnant? Sweat began to drip down my arms. The insides of my gloves were soaked. "I'm trying," I said. "Trying again." The idea that there might be a fetus just inches from the tip of my needle was almost too much to fathom. I looked at the patient's belly as my heart continued to heave.

"Just put it in the vein," someone shouted. It reminded me of those moments on the pitcher's mound when I found accuracy eluding me and fans would yell out, "Just throw strikes!" I steadied the needle and again felt for the femoral artery. I plunged the needle even deeper. Suddenly, the syringe filled with fluid and I exhaled. But the fluid was not purple. It wasn't red either. It was yellow.

"That's piss, dude," someone said. "Try again."

Had I inserted the needle so far that I'd punctured her bladder? It seemed unlikely, but I didn't know. "I can't get it," I said and quickly withdrew the needle. It was impossible to tell if I'd stabbed the uterus.

"No, no," a different voice said from behind me. "Stay."

I didn't have to turn around to know it was Baio. "Do this," he said, placing my hands in the appropriate locations like he was teaching me to play billiards. "Here . . . here and go." He took a step back from me and said, "Do it."

The woman's body was still bouncing from the CPR. I took a deep breath and plunged the large needle into her groin. Again nothing. I stared at the empty syringe as the team continued chest compressions. What was I doing wrong? I placed my hand on the groin and felt for the artery. I thought I felt something and quickly plunged the needle in yet again.

A moment later dark blood filled the syringe and the IV was in.

"He got it," Baio said to the arrest resident. Atropine, epinephrine, and dopamine quickly streamed through the IV.

He got it. I mouthed the words to myself. My heart felt like it was going to jump out of my chest. *He got it.* As the medications coursed into her body, the image of Charles McCabe and that banana peel twinkled brightly in my mind. I imagined him watching this chaotic scene unfold, encouraging us to save this young woman. I imagined Dave turning to Petrak: *He got it.*

"Come on," I said to the lifeless body. More than anything, I wanted her to live. I didn't know her, but I wanted her to be a success story, one I would remember. A moment I could build upon.

We had just passed the ten-minute mark when a nurse yelled, "We have a pulse!"

Chest compressions were held and a pulse was confirmed. "ICU. Now!" someone shouted and a path was cleared. We had just brought the woman back from the dead and I'd played an integral role. Without that large IV, the essential medications wouldn't have been given at a sufficient rate. Six of us frantically wheeled the young woman to a service elevator.

"Keep your finger on the pulse," the arrest resident said to me, placing my free hand onto her femoral artery. "If you lose that pulse, we have to restart CPR."

In the elevator, I closed my eyes to focus on the sensation of the weak, thready pulse. A minute later we burst into the ICU, where a small group of physicians stood waiting for us. While we were finding an empty room for the young woman, a thought crossed my mind: Should I tell the ICU physicians that I might have punctured her bladder? It could potentially heal on its own. I'd seen residents do far worse things to a groin. Time seemed to slow down as I considered the retreat, the microscope, and those damn Lithuanian eyebrows. Was the second-guessing inevitable? I stared at the woman's belly as we transferred her from the stretcher to an ICU bed.

"We have a pulse and we have a blood pressure," the arrest resident said as a respiratory therapist squeezed a bag of oxygen down her breathing tube. "She was asystolic for ten minutes, but we brought her back."

"Excellent," the ICU attending physician said as he put on a pair of gloves and approached the patient. "Great work. Anything else we should know?"

I shook my head.

I made my way toward the elevator, contemplating my next move. What was I doing before the arrest? I retied the drawstring on my scrubs and scratched my head. Oh, right, I had been battering a vending machine. I looked down at my scut list and the two doodles I'd drawn on it earlier in the day. One was of a pyramid and the other was of Scrooge McDuck. The scribbles recalled Peter and his legal pad, and

Denise + Peter

I came to a halt in the center of a long hallway and stared at a newly painted taupe wall. On it I imagined the heart Peter had drawn—a punctured heart, really—and Diego's words wafted into my head. *Who are you looking out for? Yourself? Your reputation? Or the patient?*

I boomeranged back into the ICU, dashing past a group of nurses to find the attending physician, who was explaining ventilator settings to a medical student. "Gotta tell you something," I said quickly. "Your new patient . . . during the arrest, it took me several tries to get the line in. I might have . . . punctured her bladder. It's possible."

I didn't care if word got around, I didn't care if I had to sit in front of advisers and explain how it could've happened. It was an accident. The attending removed his hand from the ventilator and nodded. "Okay." He frowned briefly and looked at his medical student.

"I'm sorry I didn't mention it before. I don't know why I didn't say something. I'm sorry."

The doctor put his hand on my shoulder. "Thank you for telling me."

"I'm sorry, it was an accident."

He shook his head. "It's okay. We'll take care of it." He gave me a gentle tap on the back. "Good work."

I left the ICU and headed toward the lobby to buy a bottle of water. I passed a large mirror and noticed I was a bit hunched over, perhaps still trying to catch my breath and wrap my head around the moment. *He got it.* I felt my phone buzz and read the new text message from Mark: NICE WORK DUDE!

I checked the time and realized it was almost time for my next round of HIV medications. Standing in front of the elevators, I encountered Moranis and his tour group.

"Save her?" he asked.

I nodded. "We did."

"Super!" He started to clap, and the applicants joined in.

It was an odd moment, receiving a round of gentle applause from a group of strangers. "I put in the line," I said.

Moranis smiled. "That's great!" He leaned his head toward mine and to the side and softly said, "Hey, I know you're busy, but when you get the chance, give Sam a call. He's got a few questions about his medications. Just give him a little TLC."

"Oh, sure. He wants to talk . . . to me?"

Moranis smiled. "He wants to talk to someone. And I think it should be you." As the elevator arrived, Moranis turned to the tour group and said, "Dr. McCarthy is one of our internal medicine interns, and he's doing a bang-up job. Keep up the good work, Doctor."

PART IV

31

As the days grew shorter and the winter holidays approached, I increasingly found myself thinking of Benny. It usually happened in small moments—waiting for an elevator, making a selection at a vending machine—when I had a few seconds to process just how differently the passage of time was affecting us. Through sheer repetition, I was becoming a more competent doctor. Inserting the large IV successfully had earned me a well-timed boost of confidence, as well as a public commendation from Dave at the next intern report. And the young woman's bladder had not been punctured; the fluid wasn't urine but abdominal fluid, coming from around the muscles. After that I placed four more large IVs in quick succession. With each one I burned off a bit more of the cloud that had hovered over me in the fall. I grew better at making diagnoses, more comfortable using an ophthalmoscope, and more relaxed interacting with patients. I knew I was still under a microscope, but I was no longer subjected to one-on-one meetings about my mental health. I could just show up for work and do my job.

But the changing of the calendar brought nothing for Benny. There was no silver lining to his interminable stay in the hospital. He simply waited day after day after day for a heart that might not ever come. Some days he moved up on the wait list, on others he slid down. The pogo sticking was inevitable, and Benny said he was at peace with the process. But I wasn't. There were many things to complain about in our healthcare system—the inefficiency, the barbaric hours, the waste—but his plight was gradually consuming my thoughts. Why were we doing this to him? It seemed like he was stuck in an absurdist play.

If there was one constant in our chaotic hospital, it was Benny. His name evoked one of a handful of mental images from the rotating cast of providers who cared for him: reading under fluorescent lighting, jotting in a journal, using lightweight silverware, being prodded and poked like a fledgling fire. Graciously allowing doctors, nurses, and medical students to interrupt whatever he was doing to check his vital signs, listen to his lungs, or peer into his mouth. I had often joked with Benny that while I felt like I lived in the hospital, he actually did. But by December the jokes had faded and we found ourselves talking mostly about faith and hope, formulating strategies for coping with an endless hospital stay, talking about how things might be different one day.

Our roads were diverging, and the metaphor I'd created for our simultaneous journey was breaking down. One evening in late December, when I wanted nothing more than to be home with my family, I took a break from my work and popped in to see a man whom I presumed felt the same way.

"Mr. Santos," I said as I stepped into his room. Magazines and journal entries were once again scattered across his bed, and a pair of headphones was resting above a stack of CDs on his nightstand. We never dwelled on his writings, but I knew he was documenting his interminable hospital stay. I often thought of how his meticulous penmanship stood in such contrast to the presumably messy subject matter. Several medications were dripping into his arm through a large IV that was attached to a metal pole as he watched a Knicks game.

"Come in, come in," he said, waving me toward the distressed leather chair in the corner of the room.

"What's new?" I asked.

He muted the television and shook his head. "Nothing new. Nothing new with me, nothing new with the Knicks. You?"

"Same ol' stuff," I said, taking a seat. I stared out at the Hudson River, as I had so many times, wondering if it was going to freeze over.

The river was nearly still, its dark water bleak and ominous, and I momentarily felt the urge to compare it to Benny's predicament. "Almost halfway through the year," I said. Benny wrinkled his brow, perhaps contemplating a mental calendar, before I added, "almost halfway through *intern* year."

"Right! Congratulations. You'll be running this place soon."

We both smiled. "I hope not."

Our eyes gradually drifted to the Knicks game, and I tried not to ask the question I always asked, but I couldn't resist. "Anything going on with the wait list?"

"No news is bad news," he said softly, like air being let out of a balloon.

We stared at the television impassively as I thought of something to say. I worried that my constant reminders of the wait list weren't helpful. Just because I thought about it didn't mean he needed to. Did forcing this kind man from Miami—a guy who'd spent most of his childhood on a beach—to talk about his limited, difficult life help him in any way? Probably not. I needed to change the subject.

"But I have faith," he said. "I know God has a plan."

He had said this many times before. Over time it had become clear to me just how deep Benny's faith ran. It was, strangely, the biggest chasm between us. At first, it embarrassed me; then it angered me. How could he believe that this was all part of a master plan, that a supreme being was choosing to confine him to a hospital, waiting for a heart that might not ever come? Then I came to see that, our caregiving notwithstanding, his faith was the primary thing keeping him alive. His perpetual good nature, his resilience in the face of countless near-fatal setbacks—all was built on the foundation of his belief that God would take care of him. I had to admire the intensity of his belief, even if I couldn't share it.

"It's not fair" was all I could muster.

My tired eyes drifted down from Benny's face to his light blue hospital gown, and as I zeroed in on his chest, the Bee Gees song "Stayin'

Alive" began playing in my head. What if Benny's frail heart gave out? Would I be able to lunge into action? Would I be able to bring him back to life? Could I perform chest compressions so vigorously that his ribs might crack?

"What?" he asked. "What's not fair?"

But my mind had already moved on. Our conversations were often like this—clumsy, uneven, awkward. Prolonged silence often followed an unanswered question. I routinely lost my train of thought in mid-sentence, remembering that there was something else I needed to do for a different patient on a different floor. There was a condition called ICU delirium—living in an intensive care unit can cause profound cognitive impairment—and I occasionally wondered if he had it. My sleep deprivation certainly didn't help things. We were two delirious guys, just trying to hold a conversation.

"Medicine," I said, feeling my voice tighten, "is the only place I can think of where everyone is miserable. Doctors are miserable, patients are miserable, support staff is—"

"I'm not miserable," he said. He turned his head away from the television and locked eyes with me. "Really, I'm not."

I knew he was telling the truth. But it still confounded me. When a patient yelled at me or an error was made, it was easier to think of something else—to think of Benny—and transfer the anger or disappointment in my own moment to the faceless system that had wronged him. But there was no one person to blame for his situation. Certainly not his doctors, who vigorously advocated for him at the weekly transplant meetings, not the nurses, not the organ donors, not even the administrators at the UNOS organ-sharing network, who had carefully crafted an algorithm to remove subjectivity from the allocation process. There was no one to blame, no one to silently curse. But that didn't change the way I felt. He said he wasn't miserable, but I felt that way for him.

"The whole thing is bullshit," I said under my breath. I again wondered if I'd crossed the line between patient and friend. Technically he was no longer my patient; he was just another guy stuck in the hospital over the holidays. He was more than that, though, and we both knew it.

"Well, today I am miserable," I said, looking at the clock. "I'm on hour seventeen of thirty. These shifts are insane."

Still, I felt no urge to get up. Even though I was inching my way out from under the microscope, I had not yet totally recovered from Dre's wordless departure. Calibrating my emotional investment in patients still filled me with anxiety. It was easier to live behind the wall, to stay detached, which was fine but for the lingering feeling that each time I withheld some piece of myself from my patients, I was doing them a disservice. I balanced the guilt with a rational explanation: I didn't need to relate to my patients' pain because it was all I could do to handle my own. But underneath the excuses my need to connect with patients still existed; it was a fundamental quality of the doctor I wanted to be. I suspected I was spending more time with Benny to compensate for the barricade I'd constructed for others.

"Don't know how you guys do it," he said. "I really don't."

"I'm gonna look like ass in the morning."

Benny's attention returned to the television, and I reflexively checked my pager. I felt awkward eliciting his sympathy. He didn't need to hear how long I'd be in the hospital or how tired I'd be in the morning. With all that was going on around him, I doubted he ever got a decent night of sleep. But complaining had, for so many interns, become second nature. It may even have been part of the twelve-step process toward breaking. Enthusiastic intern becomes bitter intern becomes broken intern. "Some of it's great," I added, "but some of it is rough."

Benny turned off the television, and I took this as a sign that I was allowed to vent. There was so much I wanted to say, so much of the quiet hellishness of an intern's life that I wanted to describe. Why did Benny need to be the one to hear about it? Because my colleagues already knew what it was like and people outside the hospital would never understand. But Benny Santos, professional patient, was a man apart.

"Talk to me," he said.

I took off my white coat as a symbolic gesture that I was now talking as a friend, not a physician. "So many things go into being a doctor," I said, "connecting with patients, medical knowledge, performing procedures—and on any given day you can consider yourself a failure at one of them. Or all of them." He nodded. "You can beat yourself up to the point that you're ready to quit. But on the other hand . . . at any moment you can look around and say, 'I'm better than that guy. I'm a better doctor than her.'"

"Huh."

"So much of it is mental."

"I can imagine."

"I'm sure you can."

"It's like sports," he said, pointing to his head. "All mental."

"It's like you have to trick yourself into thinking you should stick with it. And to be honest, I resent the fact that some of my buddies—the same ones who could never get into medical school—are making ungodly sums of money while Heather and I are hundreds of thousands of dollars in debt."

Benny looked away, and I realized I'd said too much. I glanced down at my scut list, embarrassed that I was complaining to someone who had so much more to complain about. It felt good to vent, but then it didn't.

"How is Heather?" he asked. "She good?"

"She's great." I didn't mention that residency had also affected my personal life. Intimacy was something that now almost had to be planned. And when we discovered that we had a night off together, it was euphoric. Otherwise it was like being in a long-distance relationship with the person you live with. I stared at Benny, lost in his big, wet, brown eyes. I knew I was talking too much. "Tell me about the Knicks," I said.

He didn't tell me about the Knicks. Instead, he clasped his hands like he was about to pray. "You guys," he said, "give me hope. Makes me feel like you're invested in me. Invested in what happens."

The comment caught me off guard. I tried to think of something significant to say. "Of course we are."

Benny shifted positions in his chair. "I meant to ask, Matt, what happened with that test?"

My mind quickly scanned all of the daily tests, both literal and figurative, and drew a blank. "What test?"

"Few weeks ago I passed you in the lobby and you said you were having a test. Or getting the results of a test. A blood test."

Oh, right. *That* test.

After I'd completed my ridiculously complex regimen of pills, a series of blood tests had been arranged to determine if I'd contracted hepatitis C or HIV. The intervening days—after the blood was collected and while the tests were being performed—had been some of the most nerve-racking of my life. I was unable to sleep, I was distracted on rounds, and if I thought too deeply about the possibility of living with HIV, I dry-heaved. I had bounded past Benny in the hospital's lobby on my way to see Banderas to learn the results.

"Right," I said. "I forgot we bumped into each other."

I briefly closed my eyes and considered what I had told Benny and what I wanted to tell him. I knew so much about him, so much about his medical history and his personal history, so much about the contours of his skin and his allergies and the unique way his heart murmured, but he knew relatively little about me. I had mentioned the needle stick in passing but hadn't told him about the HIV risk or the pills. It felt unfair to burden him with my issue when he was dealing with so much more. But maybe I should have. Isn't that what genuine friendship is actually about?

On the morning Benny was referring to, I'd woken up at 4:15 and popped out of bed knowing that my test results would be available later that day. I'd yanked a dress shirt and tie out of my closet, imagining myself as a sickly young man, a doctor with a chronic illness in need of a new wardrobe, with smaller clothes that would fit my withered frame and long-sleeved T-shirts to hide the skin abscesses that were destined to appear on my arms. I'd skipped breakfast and braced for the worst.

I'd kept my head bowed on the subway to work, silently praying that things would turn out okay. In between prayers, I'd glanced around the train for Ali—the fraudulent spiritual adviser, *my* fraudulent spiritual adviser—but I wasn't sure why. Perhaps I took comfort in familiarity; I liked the pretend powers I projected onto him. He was a sign of normalcy. At that point, I would've taken any sign that I'd be okay. If Ali was on the train, being weird, all would be right in the world.

During rounds, I had quietly counted the minutes until Employee Health opened and sprinted toward Banderas's office the moment I could excuse myself. I had nearly knocked Benny over when I turned a corner and bumped into him in the lobby.

Sitting in Benny's room on that cold night in December, I wanted to tell him about all of this, I wanted to tell him how I'd imagined Banderas rolling into work, checking his email, pulling up my test results, perhaps putting a hand to his face, wondering if he could break the bad news to me over the phone or if I needed to be told in person. I wanted to tell Benny that I could have checked the results on the computer myself but I was afraid to. I wanted to recount every moment in painstaking detail just as I'd lived it.

But when I looked into Benny's eyes, I chose not to say any of this. A man who'd been on the receiving end of so much bad news in his life didn't need a dramatic reenactment of my good news.

"Things worked out," I said.

"Oh." A smile emerged over his face. "Oh, that's wonderful. I'm so relieved for you. Whatever it was." He stood up to hug me, but the IV kept him tethered to the metal pole, so he waved me toward him. As I leaned in and extended my arms, as if on cue, my pager went off and I was summoned to the intensive care unit for an orientation session.

32

The first night on call of my rotation in the intensive care unit occurred in mid-January, as a gentle snowfall blanketed Washington Heights. I was lying on a black leather couch in the doctors' lounge, reviewing a stack of EKGs, when the door flung open.

"Nap time's over," a voice said as I pushed a banana peel off my chest and flung myself upright. "Looks like we've got some more business."

The voice belonged to my blond, floppy-haired supervisor, Don, a second-year resident who had taken over for Baio and Ashley as my medical swag coach. Among the many disorienting aspects of intern year was the constant shuffling of supervisors. Just when I became comfortable with one resident's style, I was pawned off on a new resident with a new system. The carousel of bosses meant I was exposed to all kinds of teaching philosophies, and as the year wore on, I realized just how special Baio had been. Others were excellent in their own ways—some were nimble with needles, others were master negotiators—but no one quite brought the incredible immediacy of medicine to life the way Baio had.

I had heard of Don before I had ever spoken with him. He was a bit of a cornball—a milquetoast midwesterner who loved to show cell phone pictures of his eight-month-old son—but more recently he was known around the hospital as the guy who had picked up a congenital blood vessel abnormality in a young woman after noticing a subtle difference in blood pressure readings in her arms. Word of his careful eye had spread quickly, and Don was now regarded as a master diagnostician. I suspected that he, like Baio, was someone special, and I couldn't wait to work with him. Don reinforced my belief that professional reputations could be created or destroyed with a single patient.

"New admission from the emergency room," Don said, gliding across the linoleum. His face was pinched—as if his features were rallying around the scar from his surgically repaired cleft palate—and I wasn't yet sure if he was one of those guys who would lord his sterling reputation over me. He picked up the black plastic phone and put it on speaker.

"Fellas," the voice on the other end said. It was Baio.

"My man," Don replied. "I'm here with Matt McCarthy. What you got for us?"

"Kindly give Dr. McCarthy my regards."

I moved toward the phone, took a seat in an orange plastic chair, and said, "Hey!"

"Got a young guy down here in the ED," Baio said quickly. "Nineteen-year-old morbidly obese kid with asthma coming in acutely short of breath. Labs look like shit. Chest X-ray looks like shit. I'm thinking it's . . ."

"Influenza?" Don asked.

"Oh, Don," Baio said, not nearly as impressed with Don's powers of deduction.

"Sorry, sorry," Don said, picking up a marker, "I'll shut up now."

"We're thinking viral infection with superimposed bacterial pneumonia. Probably triggered an asthma exacerbation. We might have to tube him."

"Yikes," I said softly. I hadn't heard of someone so young requiring a ventilator.

"Well, send him on up," Don said. "He'll take our last bed. ICU's full."

The conversation abruptly ended, and Don stood up and moved to a small white marker board. "Stupid mistake," he said. "Never hone in on a diagnosis so quickly. Let's make a list of the things this kid could have *other* than infection. Go."

Life in the medical intensive care unit was wildly unpredictable. Some nights we admitted up to a half dozen new, exceedingly sick, exceedingly complex patients. Working in the ICU required an advanced grasp of physiology and the ability to remain calm yet assertive while dealing with complex, terrifyingly sick patients. It was the perfect fit for a guy like Baio, but not so much for me. Patients in the ICU are often too sick to describe the events that led up to their admission, and the aim is not to cure a condition but rather to stabilize it. There isn't much red meat there for doctors who find meaning through personal connection.

Fortunately, tonight was looking relatively quiet. Our unit was nearly full and Don had put out most of the fires earlier in the evening, so we had some time to talk. He and I spent the next half hour creating a preposterously long list of what might be wrong with our new patient, until a nurse knocked on the door, poked her head in, and said, "New admission, Darryl Jenkins, is being wheeled in now."

Don dropped the marker. "Showtime."

33

I watched closely as Don examined Darryl, who was clutching his chest while gasping for air. Darryl's huge body took up the entire hospital bed. He must've weighed three hundred pounds, and yet his face was childlike—he looked like a boy trapped in a body far too large for him. And he looked like a wreck. I could hear him wheeze from across the room. Large beads of sweat dripped from his forehead down the side of his face as a nurse placed an oxygen mask on Darryl's face, and a nebulizer treatment was administered to open up his asthmatic lungs. It was jarring to see someone so young who was so sick. Don stood off to the side, fixated on Darryl's fingernails. I pulled my stethoscope out of my white coat and cleaned it off with an alcohol swab, wondering what Don was doing.

"Just going to take a quick listen," I said to Darryl as I tapped his upper back. "Need to listen to your lungs." He closed his eyes, failing to acknowledge my comment.

As I leaned in, Don said, "Stop." He was holding Darryl's left hand, shining a penlight onto the middle fingernail. "Look at this, Matt. What do you see?"

I withdrew the stethoscope and inched toward the outstretched arm. "What?" I asked.

"What do you see?" Don asked again. "Describe it to me."

It looked like a normal fingernail, perhaps slightly shorter than average. "Looks a little short," I said. "Maybe he was biting it?" I looked up at Darryl's round face; his eyes were still closed, and he was generating quick, shallow breaths. "Understandable, considering the circumstances." Two more nurses entered the room and administered more nebulizer treatments.

Don shook his head. "No." He brought the limp hand up toward his eyeballs. "Look here."

I stretched my neck and closely studied the nail. "I'm not sure I see anything." As I took the hand and held it in my own, Darryl began a vigorous coughing spell and pulled away.

"Look at the curvature of the nail bed," Don said. "It's called clubbing."

"I've heard of it," I said, enthusiastically recalling a patient on the infectious disease service who'd had the condition as a result of chronic lung disease. "I've actually seen it before. But I didn't see it here."

"It's subtle," Don said, "but it's there."

"Huh." Not only did I miss it but I wouldn't have thought to look for it.

"The question is why."

Before I could answer, Don moved to Darryl's feet, pulling off his socks to examine his toes. From there, he went behind the bed to inspect Darryl's scalp. Then he plunged his hands into Darryl's vast armpits. Last, after he'd examined every possible inch of our new patient, he listened to Darryl's lungs. His approach to the physical exam recalled the way Baio had taught me to read a chest X-ray, starting from the periphery. "He's gonna need a ventilator," Don said. "Let's go put in some orders."

After the orders were in, Don called in a team of anesthesiologists, and I looked on as they tunneled a breathing tube into Darryl's throat. After the ventilator was switched on, we retreated to the doctors' lounge.

Don assumed his position at the marker board and said, "Asthma is treated in a stepwise fashion based on pulmonary function. Walk me through those steps."

I tried to shake the image of Darryl—the flabby arms, the swollen lips forming a seal around the breathing tube, the large IV disappearing somewhere below his enormous belly—and grabbed a can of soda from a miniature refrigerator in the corner of the room. As Don pointed the marker at me, the phone rang.

"Bad news, gentlemen." Baio's voice emanated through the speakerphone. "Looks like I got another one down here for you."

Baio was working a twelve-hour overnight shift in the emergency room, assigning patients to various floors and medical teams. We all had to spend two weeks working as ER physicians to see how the other half lived, and most of my colleagues loathed the experience. Quickly triaging an endless stream of patients in the emergency room was remarkably different from what we usually did, which was to care for a confined panel of about a dozen patients within the hospital.

"Sorry," Don said, still standing, "you know we don't have any beds. The ICU is full."

"It's a frequent flier," Baio replied, referring to oft-hospitalized patients. "Honestly should go to the CCU, but they're full."

"We're full, too," Don said firmly.

"It's this guy Benny Santos. McCarthy knows him."

I nearly spat out my soda. "What's he doing in the emergency room?" I asked.

"The CCU sent him home a few days ago," Baio said. "Told him he could just wait for the heart at home. But he looks sick as shit right now."

"Fuck." At my last count, Benny had been living in the hospital for seven months; I couldn't believe they'd just sent him home. And without telling me? How did I not know about this? In truth, there was no reason to tell me. I was more his friend than his physician. I was no longer caring for him in the CCU, and there was no reason to send out a press release, no need to inform an intern like me. His cardiologists must have decided that Benny had fallen so low on the waiting list that he could simply wait at home. Or perhaps his heart had regained some strength. Maybe he didn't *need* to be hospitalized anymore. Maybe he didn't even need a transplant.

I shook my head. There were many things I was unsure of, but I knew he needed the transplant. I'd seen just how quickly illness could strike him. One afternoon we'd be watching Judge Judy admonish a man for failing to pay child support and the next Benny would be intubated, made chemically numb by anesthetics so a breathing tube could keep him alive. He could flash at any moment and should've died a dozen times. Or more.

I wondered what it had been like for Benny to be dismissed so suddenly, to unexpectedly walk outside and breathe fresh air. Perhaps it didn't feel so sudden for him. I thought of a wrongly convicted inmate being set free. They really just sent Benny home? Why didn't he tell me?

We had often joked about grabbing lunch someday "on the outside," somewhere far, far away from Columbia—somewhere that served normal food and had real utensils. I never thought that day would come, but it now appeared it had come and gone. Benny had been released and now he was back, sitting in our emergency room. And based on Baio's judgment, he was very sick and needed to be in an intensive care unit. Contemplating what Benny must have gone through—the relief of being discharged, the pain of realizing it was only temporary—was dizzying.

"No room," Don said loudly. "We can't take him. I'm sorry. The ICU is full."

"Make room," Baio said.

I stared at the phone, waiting for Don to say something. Baio knew how tenuous Benny's health was. Did Don? There was tremendous pressure on the emergency room physicians to quickly triage their sickest patients. Baio was expected to see a new patient every twenty minutes during his ER stint; one train wreck of a patient with no place to go could lead to a bottleneck and a preposterously long wait for others.

"Look," Baio said, "I know how it works up there. There's gotta be somebody you can bump."

Intensive care residents like Don were under similar pressure. ICU beds were at a premium, and patients on the mend were transitioned out of the unit and to the general hospital ward the moment they were ready. But sending someone out prematurely could lead to a bounce-back, a dreaded situation in which the patient returned to the ICU less than twenty-four hours after discharge. Don put his hand over the speaker and whispered to me, "We could put Santos in the corner pocket."

I shook my head. "No!" I whispered back.

There was one room in the ICU, in the near right corner, where patients reportedly went to die. Don told me he'd never seen someone make it out of the corner pocket alive. Everyone knew it was just a coincidence, but practicing medicine had made some of us, including my pod mates, increasingly superstitious. There was no way we were putting Benny there.

"We'll see what we can do," Don said. "We won't leave you hanging."

"Like I said, still trying to get Santos to the CCU," Baio said. "I'll talk to Diego and let you know. Later, fellas."

Don looked up from the phone and took a deep breath. "Looks like we're in for a wild night. Let's run the list before shit gets crazy."

My mind was lingering on something Baio had said about Benny: *McCarthy knows him.* How did he know that? Did he remember that we'd cared for Benny together months ago, or was this part of my reputation? Did people know that I popped in to chat with him? Was Don the master diagnostician while I was just Benny's buddy?

I pulled out my list, scanned the dozen ICU patients, and prepared to take down my marching orders. My eyes were heavy, and the night was only in its infancy. "Let's divide and conquer," Don said. "First up, Mr. Jones, forty-one-year-old with HIV here with PCP pneumonia. Did you review his chest X-ray?"

I barely heard him. My thoughts were still with Benny in the emergency room, presumably gasping for air or clutching his chest. I needed to be professional. I needed to focus on the patients in the ICU, and Benny was in good hands with Baio. I couldn't play favorites. I needed to be a utilitarian, providing the greatest benefit for the greatest number of patients, and that meant focusing on the task at hand, not the guy in the emergency room. I tried to remove the mental image of Benny from my mind. But how?

"Matt," Don said loudly, "did you review the X-ray?"

"Yes. Yes, I did." Lung tissue had been replaced by air bubbles called blebs that looked like tiny, innumerable blisters. "Never seen anything like it."

"We have to be prepared for the worst," Don said. "What are you going to do if Mr. Jones's blood pressure suddenly tanks tonight?"

"Fluids," I said, recalling Baio's introductory lesson on shock. It was as vivid now as it had been months ago. "Probably sepsis."

"Maybe," Don said, "or . . . ?"

I had gotten better at these little give-and-takes; Don was good at them, and I hoped I would be, too, someday. "Heart failure?" I offered.

"His lungs! They're filled with blebs that are just waiting to burst. And if one does, he's screwed."

"Right," I said, tossing my empty soda can into the trash. "The blebs."

"So, Dr. McCarthy, a bleb bursts at three A.M. and I'm taking a piss. What are you going to do about it?"

This is precisely what made intern year so difficult. Just when you developed some confidence, just when you thought you'd mastered a critical mass of knowledge, you were thrown a curveball. Something you've never seen before that set everything back to square one. It wasn't my fault—it was impossible to see every medical condition in the first six months—but it bothered me. Another piece of the canvas of my mind was about to be splattered with paint. "I'm not sure."

Don put his arm around me. "It's okay, big guy, that's why I'm here." He stood up at the marker board. "Tension pneumothorax. His chest will fill up with air but he can't breathe any of it. He'll suffocate in minutes. Or less."

I started scribbling. In medical school I had read about blebs and tension pneumothorax, and I had memorized the ways to treat it. But this was different. Every time I moved to a new floor, I had to familiarize myself not only with new supervisors and nurses but also with new equipment. Even if I knew *how* to treat tension pneumothorax, I might not know where to find the equipment on my own. Every floor had a different supply room and a different way of arranging its inventory.

"Your job," Don said as he ran his hands through his hair, "should you choose to accept it, is to stick a needle in Mr. Jones's chest, just a few inches below the collarbone, to let the air out."

"Got it," I said, recalling the instructional video on *The New England Journal of Medicine* website. It was a tricky procedure to perform, and I hoped I'd be able to do it properly. I wondered if these medical maneuvers would ever become second nature, if my pulse would eventually cease to race at the thought of inserting a needle into another human. I hoped not. I thought of the Asian doctor I'd seen many months ago, submerging a large needle into the lining of someone's heart. These outlandish, lifesaving interventions were unnatural, and the day they became mundane would be the day I lost a bit of my humanity.

"Yes. It's a shame," Don said. "This all could've been prevented if Mr. Jones had just taken his HIV meds." I closed my eyes and thought: *Not as easy as you think.*

"Bed ten, Ms. Hansen, is a potential bump," Don said.

"Is she the one from Canada?" I asked. At times it was difficult to differentiate the ICU patients; most were sedated and intubated, draped under gowns or special machinery to augment their core body temperature. I hated to admit it, but a lot of the patients in the intensive care unit looked alike.

"Yeah," Don said, jotting something on his hand. "A few days ago she was found unconscious in her living room by a neighbor. The guys in the ER couldn't get a central line into her femoral vein so they went straight into her shin." We both winced; the interosseous approach was preposterously painful, but there had been no other option for giving her a rapid infusion of medications. "She's still full code, but her healthcare proxy just arrived. I think it's her daughter. See if you can get her to change to comfort measures only."

Comfort measures only meant we were effectively throwing in the towel; aggressive attempts at resuscitation would be over and life-prolonging interventions like dialysis would be withdrawn. Most people hadn't thought about what medical interventions they'd want if the unthinkable happened, and even fewer had assigned someone to carry out their wishes. Family members were often left to confront these decisions for the first time when a loved one landed in the ICU. Overwhelmed with heartbreaking decisions, many healthcare proxies simply asked that we "do everything." But this wasn't always in the best interests of the patients. It could lead to expensive, futile procedures and merely prolong the inevitable. Conveying this with tact was a skill. With no textbook to provide guidance, interns were left to figure out how to lead these discussions in much the way we learned anything—through observation, practice, and occasional failure.

"Okay," I said, "I missed the discussion on rounds. Did we decide that Ms. Hansen's chances of recovery are nonexistent?"

"She's dying. She's suffering. No one in the family wants to acknowledge that. They keep saying 'do everything' because it helps them sleep at night."

The word *suffering* recalled my conversation with Dr. Phillips. He had left Columbia for another hospital shortly after I'd discharged his patient safely. Word came back that he was going to a nonteaching hospital where he wouldn't have to deal with interns. "Tough spot," I said, wondering how I'd handle things if my mother was in the intensive care unit and I had to make decisions on her behalf. I also thought of Benny. If her family decided to withdraw life-prolonging measures, Marlene Hansen would no longer need to be in an ICU. There would be a spot for Benny in our unit and I could go down to the ER to retrieve him myself.

"It's not a tough spot," Don said. "It's outrageous that the family is doing this to their mother. And our hands are tied."

"Are they?" I didn't have a solution, but I had learned from Baio to ask more questions when answers were proving elusive. "Can't we just say enough is enough?" I asked. "I mean, who's running the show here?"

"Better go talk to the daughter now," Don said. "If Hansen becomes comfort measures only then we can send her out of the unit. We'll have room for that second patient in the ER you know."

Was he hinting at my emotional attachment to Benny? The idea made me uncomfortable. "Everyone definitely agreed on rounds that she should be comfort measures only?"

"Yes. She suffered a massive heart attack, which deprived her brain of oxygen for so long that she's brain-dead. Her kidneys are failing. Soon she'll need dialysis. And the neurologists came by and confirmed there's no brain activity."

"Huh."

"We could keep her alive," Don said, "but to what end?"

"Okay. I've only done a couple of these goals-of-care discussions. How, uh, do you usually go about it?"

"As it stands, if Ms. Hansen's heart stops we're supposed to do CPR. Ribs crack, the whole deal. Just try to convey that scene as clearly and vividly as possible. It's one thing to do it to a thirty-year-old. But this woman is brain-dead." He put his hand on my shoulder. "There's no right way to have this conversation. Don't tell them what to do; help them figure out what's best."

I imagined uncooked spaghetti cracking under my palms and again asked myself what I would I do if my mother were in this situation. Could I live with myself if I pulled the plug and there had been even a sliver of a chance of recovery? And would I do it based on the recommendations of an intern? People occasionally recover from a vegetative state, don't they? I was certain that someone at some point in history had recovered. Right?

"Don't look so stressed," Don said as he scooped a handful of Goldfish crackers into his mouth. "This'll be good practice."

Was there any other job, I wondered, where practicing involved telling someone she was better off letting her mother die? It sure seemed like the real deal to me. But perhaps I was approaching the conversation the wrong way. Was there a way to offer comfort to Ms. Hansen's daughter while conveying that all hope was lost? I began testing out opening lines, imagining how I wanted the dialogue to play out. This kind of story line never appeared on any sitcom or drama that I was familiar with. I closed the door to the lounge and made the slow walk toward Ms. Hansen's room, vigorously grinding my teeth along the way.

34

"I'm not a doctor," Ingrid Hansen said, sitting in an orange plastic chair next to her mother. "I'm still trying to wrap my brain around what happened." I brought another chair into the room and took a seat. "She was fine a week ago." Her green eyes darted back and forth as she stared at the floor; Ingrid wore knee-high leather boots and a nose ring and couldn't have been a day over twenty-one. She took a sip from a large cup of coffee and reached for her scarf, which was resting on her purse. From the looks of things, she hadn't slept in days.

I tried to calibrate how close it was appropriate to sit. What was the right way to do this? I slid my chair a few inches closer to Ingrid, and she looked on as I briefly scanned her mother's ventilator settings. "Tell me what your understanding is thus far," I said, parroting a phrase Don often used with families.

"I don't know," she said. "Someone found her. She had a heart attack, she had a stroke. She won't wake up."

As with so many of my patients and their families, I tried to imagine what their home life was like. Was she close with her mother? Did they talk on the phone? Did they fight? Did Ingrid truly understand what her mother would want in this nightmare scenario?

"She had a massive heart attack," I said, measuring my words. "Blood wasn't able to pump to her brain. We don't know exactly how long she was down." I fought the urge to look away when Ingrid's lower lip began to tremble, and again I thought of my own mother. "She suffered profound brain damage," I went on. "There is no brain activity."

"Oh . . . God."

I could feel a part of myself shutting down as Ingrid's eyes welled with tears. It had become a slightly habitual reaction since Dre, when I was faced with such raw suffering, but now, with my health in the clear and my position at the hospital feeling more secure, I knew I needed to break myself of it. I took Ingrid's soft hand in mine and searched for words as ventilator and blood pressure alarms blared in the background. My hand was cold, and I could tell it wasn't providing comfort. She flinched when my palm touched hers and I thought she was going to pull away, but she didn't. Her lower lip continued to tremble. When she closed her eyes, a tear dripped down her cheek. "We have the option to scale back." I struggled to find the right balance between staying empathetic and not crying myself.

She took a deep breath and dabbed her cheeks with her scarf. "Is she suffering?"

"That is a concern, yes."

"I don't understand."

We sat in silence as I considered my words. I wasn't sure I was handling this conversation the right way, but it didn't feel like the wrong way either. I felt my pager buzz and fought the urge to throw it against the wall. "Sometimes there's no rhyme or reason," I said softly.

"I just don't . . . How can she be suffering if there's no brain activity?"

I did not have an answer. And then, a moment of terror. What if this was the moment Baio had been talking about—a time when I was instructed to do something that I shouldn't? Something that was wrong. "There are certain things we know," I said. "We know that—"

As the words trickled out, I became less certain. During rounds, when the team had discussed Marlene Hansen, I had been called away to transport a patient to the MRI scanner. I hadn't been there to hear just how dire her case was. It was clear from reading the notes of other physicians that a consensus had been reached that she no longer needed to be in an ICU, but I was technically relying on secondhand information. I was basing my conversation with Ingrid on the opinion of Don and experts whom I barely knew—medical consultants who had only met Marlene Hansen a day or two ago. What if they were wrong? What if I deferred this conversation until morning, when the rest of the team was available? What if that caused Benny to remain stuck in the emergency room because no ICU or CCU beds were available?

"I'll do what you want," Ingrid said softly, removing her hand from mine.

"You shouldn't do what I want. And difficult as it may be, you shouldn't do what you want. You should do what your mother would want. Have you ever discussed what she might want in this situation?"

"No."

"But you are her healthcare proxy?"

She nodded. "She doesn't have anyone else."

"There is something called comfort measures only. We won't draw blood, we won't poke her with needles. We'll make her comfortable."

"I thought she couldn't feel anything."

"Right."

"If she gets an infection, would you give her antibiotics?"

I wasn't sure. I hadn't even been present for the discussion on rounds about what was appropriate. Ingrid took her mother's hand and kissed it. "I don't want her to suffer," she said. "I trust you. Just show me what I need to sign."

I closed my eyes and bit my lip. I had been sent in to carry out a mission—to get Marlene Hansen out of the ICU—but it was clear that I didn't have all of the necessary information. Maybe in a few hours I would, after I'd reviewed all of the notes from other doctors, but at that moment I wasn't sure about very basic things like whether we'd provide antibiotics.

I mostly believed I was doing the right thing, but I wasn't certain. It was impossible to know everything—I'd never know how to read an electroencephalogram, I'd never be the one to perform dialysis; those were jobs for experts in neurology and nephrology, and I had to trust them. If they felt Marlene Hansen had no hope of recovery, they were probably right. But what if I'd met Marlene instead of Benny? What if she was the patient trapped in the hospital—the one I visited day after day—the one I felt an emotional attachment to? Would this conversation have played out differently?

I wasn't sure.

A moment later, I returned with the paperwork and handed Ingrid a pen. As she signed her name, I imagined myself taking the pen back, tearing up the papers, and telling Don that Ingrid wasn't entirely sure what her mother would want. That was the truth of it. With space available, it seemed prudent to keep Marlene Hansen in the ICU until Ingrid figured it out. But what purpose would that serve? Was Ingrid going to suddenly recall some distant conversation with her mother about her end-of-life wishes? Was she going to remember that Mom actually wanted to be kept alive at all costs for as long as possible, even if she was brain-dead? The reality was that Don had a better grasp on how to keep the flow of traffic moving in the hospital; allowing emotions to get involved would introduce subjectivity. And subjectivity could screw things up for all of the other patients.

I kept my mouth shut and let her sign the papers.

"Nice work," Don said as I leaned over a filing cabinet and placed the paperwork into Ms. Hansen's chart. "We'll send her out in a few hours."

"Few?"

"They got a bed for Benny in the CCU."

I jolted upright. "What? So Hansen can stay?" I felt like I had been punched in the gut. Don took a bite out of a tuna sandwich and patted me on the shoulder. "Hospital doesn't function when we're at capacity, Matt. Gotta have a bed available if there's an arrest on the floor. Hansen needs to go. This is a no-brainer."

"Gotcha," I said softly.

He inhaled the remainder of his sandwich. "Get something to eat and then let's do a vitals check on the unit. There's more tuna in the lounge." And with that he headed down the hall, looking like a man who knew much more than I did.

35

It was approaching 3:00 A.M., the witching hour, when my body temperature inexplicably plummeted and the pace of work finally calmed down. Or exploded. We never knew. On a quiet night, it was the ideal time to throw on a sweatshirt and pick a supervisor's brain, catch up on paperwork, or prepare for the firing squad of morning rounds. On a disastrous night—one in which there were simultaneous cardiac arrests or a half dozen new admissions—3:00 A.M. was the time when you daydreamed about business school or working as a medical consultant for a hedge fund.

The ER sending Benny to the CCU meant we had dodged a bullet. There would be time to talk, time to check labs and vital signs, time to process the matrix of data and tidy up the unit before the rest of our team arrived at dawn. And maybe, if we were lucky, there would be time for Don to impart some wisdom. I attempted to nudge him in that direction.

"I heard about that diagnosis you made," I said. "Takayasu's arteritis. Very impressive."

Don grinned. "Attention to detail, my friend."

"There are so many details."

"Key is figuring out which ones are important. That's what intern year is about. They call them *vital* signs for a reason." I noted a hint of swagger in his voice. "I was just heads-up."

"I'll say."

He ran his hands through his blond hair. "They asked me to give a talk about it to the department. Can you believe that? What the hell do I know?"

I shrugged. Beneath Don's glimmer of swagger was vulnerability. I'd seen it when Baio had called him out on the phone. It occurred to me that we were all wrestling with some form of impostor syndrome, unable to internalize and appreciate our own accomplishments. There was always someone more impressive, someone who could make you look foolish if they really wanted to. Underneath the glimmering personas, some of us—including me and the women in my pod—secretly worried that we didn't deserve to be doctors, we didn't deserve to hold life in our hands, we weren't the ones who should be leading complex discussions about comfort measures and vegetative states. The key to residency was figuring out ways to ignore those feelings without turning into a monster.

"On second thought," Don said, "let's hold off on the vital signs. Get some food and grab a few minutes of sleep if you can. You just know the ED is teeing someone up for us."

He pulled out his cell phone and showed me several pictures of his son. The kid was crying in every one, but Don was beaming.

"You sure?" I asked. I was wide awake—stress was a remarkable stimulant—but Axel's axiom wafted into my head: *When you can sleep, sleep.*

"Couch is all yours."

In my six months at Columbia, I had observed two types of interns—those who couldn't sleep on call and those who desperately needed at least a few moments of shut-eye during the thirty-hour shift. I fell into the latter category; just eight minutes of sleep and I felt reasonably refreshed. By contrast, after a sleepless night I looked, as one colleague put it, "like someone vomited on dog shit."

I had been snoozing for two glorious hours when a brown paper bag dropped on my chest with breakfast. "How was the night?" Lalitha asked, pushing my legs off of the end of the couch. "Lounge is a mess."

"Not horrible."

Her appearance meant I'd survived the night. *Hallelujah*. She patted my thigh with an old *Us Weekly* and shook her head. "I can't believe you have a subscription to this."

I grabbed the magazine from her. "How else am I going to know Candace Cameron just lost twenty-two pounds?"

Lalitha and I made it a point to engage in conversational nonsense for a few minutes every day before the sun rose and the storm of work and morning rounds rolled in. Our lives together were so intense, so structured, so stressful, that it felt good to talk about something other than our critically ill patients.

We all struggled with the weight of our work, but having the occasional dopey conversation was a reminder that we weren't simply using each other to get through the day. We were normal people who could engage in idle chitchat. But because our personal lives were so limited—the rare off day was often spent catching up on sleep—we rarely had normal things to talk about. Celebrity gossip became linguistic currency, something we could bring up when we needed to disengage from medicine. For me, the levity of the tabloids helped balance out the tragedy of watching people die day after day.

Lalitha scanned Candace Cameron's new figure and pulled out a compact and brush from her bag.

"Did anyone ever tell you," I said, as I watched her groom, "that you look like Rudy from *The Cosby Show*?"

She rolled her eyes. "Did anyone ever tell you that you look like Pat Sajak?"

"Pat's a national treasure."

"Sajak crossed with ALF crossed with Chandler from *Friends*. When he was on drugs."

Don entered the lounge, and we sat upright. "At ease, Doctors."

"What'd you do to Matt overnight?" Lalitha asked. "Looks like a truck hit him."

I parted my hair, held the magazine over my face with my right hand, and flipped her off with my left. These little moments brought us closer.

Don shook his head. "Gotta say I love working with you two. Get along better than anyone I know."

"It's because I'm afraid of her," I deadpanned.

"He is definitely afraid of me."

"How could I not be?"

The door burst open, and the nurse manager poked her head in and calmly said, "Jones is crashing."

I dropped the magazine and grabbed Lalitha. This was the scenario Don had prepared me for: Mr. Jones, the man with the unusual lungs, had dropped his blood pressure. I felt a surge of adrenaline. "Let's do this," I said, feeling momentarily like Baio. The transition from goofball to physician was instantaneous.

"Blebs?" Lalitha asked as we bounded out of the lounge. She was a step quicker than I was. Her ponytail sashayed from side to side like a broom as we blew down the corridor past Ingrid Hansen, who was staring blankly out a window.

As we entered Jones's room, the first thing I noticed was a large window at the head of the bed. A container ship could be seen in the distance, floating south down the Hudson. The room—with its khaki walls, framed Impressionist artwork, and muted television—was oddly quiet. I was accustomed to a cacophony of alarms blaring whenever I encountered a patient in distress, but this room was silent. I imagined myself as the second-year resident, about to lead Lalitha through a resuscitation.

ABC, ABC

A nurse increased the amount of supplemental oxygen as I turned to Lalitha and announced, "Please assess the patient's—"

"Tension pneumothorax," she said quickly. "We need to decompress." She reached for two butterfly needles as I felt for a pulse. Mr. Jones's eyes were closed and he was gasping for air.

"Got a pulse," I said firmly. I stared at the man's heaving chest, relieved that I didn't need to start CPR. His ribs would have snapped with the first thrust of my palms. Jones was suffering from end-stage AIDS and pneumonia; he was emaciated, weighing less than one hundred pounds, and his cheeks were sunken in. His arms were like two Wiffle ball bats, flailing as he gasped for air. As I estimated his heart rate—it was well over one hundred beats per minute—I pictured myself doing chest compressions on this frail man, and I imagined one of the shattered ribs piercing through his heart like a warm knife through butter.

Don hung back and watched. Standing next to him, in what momentarily seemed like a mirage, was Baio. Instead of going home after his night shift, he'd come to the ICU to check on Darryl Jenkins. They both folded their arms. Part of being a strong supervisor is knowing when to let your intern take the lead, and this was apparently one of those times. Mr. Jones's eyes bulged as he squirmed in bed, panting for air. I took a deep breath. Lalitha and I were on our own.

"Have you done one of these before?" she asked as we hovered over the patient. "Needle in the chest?"

"I watched the video last night," I said, feeling like an actor in a commercial saying, "No, I'm not a doctor, but I did stay in a Holiday Inn Express last night."

"Good enough." She felt for the man's left clavicle. "I've done one. Just do what I do." She tilted her head toward his right clavicle and handed me a needle that had been attached to rubber tubing. Lalitha plunged the needle into Mr. Jones's chest and turned to me. "Go."

I felt for the landmark on my side and with my left hand thrust the needle deep into the man's meager chest. In my right hand I held the rubber tubing that was attached to the needle. Don and Baio sidled up behind us and peered over my shoulder. I waited for a gust of air, but there was nothing. "I thought a rush of air was supposed to come out," I said, "if a bleb really burst."

Lalitha and I looked at each other nonplussed as Mr. Jones continued to gasp for oxygen. Don and I hadn't discussed a Plan B. I readjusted the needle and waited for something to happen, but nothing did. I waited for Baio to say something encouraging—*you can do this*—but he just stood behind me with his arms folded and his mouth shut.

Beads of sweat gathered above my lip as Mr. Jones writhed in his bed and his blood pressure continued to plummet. Two nurses entered the room; one quickly injected a medication into the man's arm while another checked vital signs. ABC, I said to myself. He had an airway, he was breathing, and he had circulation. What was next? I was watching a man suffocate and I wasn't sure what to do. Intubation? I readjusted the needle a third time. Nothing.

I looked at Lalitha and she looked at Don. We would need to intubate him if things didn't turn around quickly. He'd also need a large IV in his groin if his blood pressure dropped again. After what felt like an eternity but was actually ten or twenty seconds, Baio handed Lalitha and me a small Styrofoam cup filled with water. I was about to take a sip when he grabbed it and said, "No." I looked at Lalitha, who had placed the tubing into the cup, and I followed her lead. Again, nothing.

I readjusted the needle a fourth time and with Baio's gentle prompting, dropped the plastic tubing into the cup of water. We both peered into my cup, which was now bubbling vigorously, and smiled. "There it is."

Air rushed out of Mr. Jones's thorax and into my cup. It was a moment straight out of *MacGyver,* not an instructional video. How did Baio come up with this stuff? I felt the muscles in my face relax just slightly. Lalitha nodded and glanced at her watch. Minutes later, Mr. Jones was breathing comfortably.

"Well done, Dr. McCarthy," Baio said, as he headed toward the exit sign. "Amazing things are indeed happening here."

36

"Not good," Benny said the next morning in the CCU. "Not good at all."

He'd lost more weight and was now using the webbed, throbbing accessory muscles of his neck to breathe. After reviving Mr. Jones in the ICU, I spent the next few hours presenting our new cases on rounds and stumbled, punch-drunk, into my apartment around noon, roughly thirty-one hours after I'd left it. When I woke up, it was 5:00 A.M. the following day. Ninety minutes later and I was standing at the foot of Benny's bed in the CCU, watching him struggle for air. His breathing wasn't as dire as Mr. Jones's—the respirations were labored, like those of a chain-smoker with emphysema—but if Benny's condition worsened, it might soon become similar. I cringed at the thought of plunging a needle under his clavicle, watching air rush into a Styrofoam cup.

"Hang in there," I said, taking a seat at the edge of his bed. We both knew time was running out—the man needed a damn heart. His legs were swollen, filled with fluid from his toes to his knees, and his jugular veins were visibly pulsing. Fluid was collecting in places it shouldn't be—I didn't have to look under his gown to know that his scrotum was probably twice its normal size—all because his heart couldn't do its job. Soon it would fill up his lungs, slowly drowning him from the inside. Benny was scared and so was I.

"Talk to me," he said. "What's new?"

My mind hopscotched across the events of the past couple of weeks; I was due back in the ICU for rounds in just a few minutes. "Why didn't you tell me you'd been discharged?" I asked. I had no right to feel slighted, but I did.

He shook his head. "I know you're a busy guy."

"You obviously don't have to tell me, but—"

"Next time I'll tell you."

Once again I felt like I was awkwardly straddling the line between physician and friend. "Let's make a deal," I said, "either one of us gets admitted to the hospital, we'll tell the other one."

"Ha. Deal."

We shook hands just as my pager went off, and I again resisted the urge to throw it against a wall. It seemed like the thing had a sensor, an organ capable of identifying important moments and interrupting them. "I really hate this thing."

"You look different," Benny said. Again our conversation was clumsy, bouncing from one unfinished thought to the next. I considered how significantly Benny's appearance had changed from when I'd met him on my first day as a doctor, but I said nothing. He was gaunt and his limbs were thin; he was a far cry from the vibrant man I'd first seen on the stationary bicycle.

"I put on some weight," I said, tugging at some loose flesh. "Somehow it all went to my neck."

"Hmm . . . That's not it."

"Bags under my eyes?"

"Nope."

"Bereft of—"

"You look older. That's what it is."

"I feel older." A week earlier I'd squealed in horror in my bathroom after acknowledging a tiny patch of gray hair. "I've accepted my fate," I said lightly. "I'll be bald by spring."

"I'm just messing with you," Benny said. He pressed a button on the side of his bed and asked for assistance. A moment later, a respiratory therapist appeared with an oxygen tank and a long, thin plastic tube that she placed under his nostrils.

"You're gonna get that fuckin' heart," I said. It was the only thing I could think of when I was in his presence. I didn't believe it, but I said it.

"Probably need a liver, too."

"And liver. You're getting the liver."

"Also need a noodle," he said, pointing at his head. "If you got one to spare."

He flashed a grin and shifted his eyes toward a picture of his wife and daughter on his nightstand. Why had I never seen them during visiting hours? Would one of them serve as his healthcare proxy? There were many probing questions that I had asked Benny, but I'd avoided this topic. Why? I suppose because I wanted to stay positive. I didn't want to venture into what would likely be an uncomfortable conversation about his absentee family. Maybe they were still in Miami.

But it wasn't just family that was absent. Throughout all these months I'd never once seen Benny with a visitor. How could someone so personable be without anyone from the outside for support? Maybe he did have visitors and I'd missed them, but that seemed unlikely. I peeked in on him at all sorts of hours, and he was always alone. Perhaps his network of friends and family simply got tired of visiting. Or tired of hearing that there was no news to report.

Did he have a dark past like Sam, my primary care patient with the criminal record? Impossible. "I'll be on the lookout for a noodle," I said as I stood up to leave. "Gotta get back to the ICU."

"Say a prayer for me," he said as oxygen began to flow from the tank into his nose. I paused, perhaps a moment too long. "Just say a prayer for me."

As I left Benny's room and hopped down a flight of stairs to the medical ICU, I ran through the questions I wanted to ask Darryl Jenkins, who, hours earlier, had been weaned from a ventilator. I wanted to see if I could connect with him—to find out if I could figure out why he had gotten so sick—while remaining emotionally detached from him. It was a fine balance, and I wasn't sure I could pull it off, but I figured it wouldn't be nearly as nerve-racking as breaking the news to Ingrid Hansen. Picking my spots with patients like this seemed both smart and a bit cowardly; how could I hedge with some and not others? The important thing, I told myself, was pushing forward, even with an imperfect plan. It would be the only way to move beyond the hesitation Dre had instilled in me, to let my guard down in a tactful yet meaningful way to get patients to trust me the way they trusted Jim O'Connell.

Darryl was one of the few patients in the unit capable of speaking, and I wasn't sure when I'd get another chance to work on my bedside manner in the ICU. Questions bounced around my head as I approached the double doors of the unit:

Could Darryl reveal some trigger or some aura that had preceded his respiratory collapse?
Why was he so profoundly and disturbingly obese?
Did he get a flu shot?

The tube had just been dislodged from Darryl's trachea, so speaking was going to be uncomfortable. I had to prioritize my questions and tried to determine if it was better to ask one or two open-ended questions or a number of yes/no questions. I wasn't sure.

"Big day," Don said, as he did every morning when I entered the ICU. His predawn arrival served as a reminder that my second year of residency would be no picnic. The hours would be just as long, and I'd have the added pressure of supervising an intern.

"Let's do it," I said, before giving him a rather inept high five and heading toward Darryl's room. It always took me a moment to adjust to the relentless braying of alarms in the ICU. On a good day, it was like dance music and I bopped from one room to the next as I made my morning rounds. On a bad day, it reminded me of honking car horns in rush-hour traffic. Today the bleating was faintly reminiscent of German prog rock, and I couldn't tell which way the day was headed.

"I'm hoping you could give me a moment of your time," I said, as I took a seat in a small chair by Darryl's bed. "I have a bunch of questions and I know you just got the tube out."

He nodded and gave a soft grunt.

"I think we can help prevent a future attack if we know more about you," I said.

He pulled a blanket up to his nose and closed his eyes. My eyes drifted to his hands and the curvature of his fingernails.

"Could you walk me through what happened the night you got sick?"

I already knew a fair amount about Darryl from the medical records that had been generated by the team of emergency room physicians who'd stabilized him before he arrived in the ICU. But there were still some holes in the story.

I knew that obesity did not run in the Jenkins family. I knew that when he was an adolescent, Darryl's mother had taken him to a specialist and the diagnosis of Prader-Willi syndrome—a condition in which genes from chromosome 15 are not expressed properly, causing a chronic feeling of hunger that often leads to life-threatening obesity—had been entertained. When it was determined that there was no genetic mutation to account for his unfortunate physique, Darryl sank into depression. And that depression, more than any other issue, dominated his life.

I had learned from his medical records that before he came to our unit, Darryl had noticed a twinge in his throat. A few hours later, he developed the telltale wheeze of an acute asthma exacerbation. But this time, his inhaler provided minimal relief. In the early evening, when his eyes began to feel like sandpaper and his breathing became labored, he called his mother from his dorm room. But there was no answer. So he called a taxi and was driven to the nearest hospital.

In the Columbia emergency room a short while later, a yellow sticker was slapped on the top of his chart and he was given an oxygen tank. Darryl was too large for a wheelchair, so he was placed on a stretcher and wheeled across the ER to have a chest X-ray. As soon as the image was uploaded, it was reviewed by Baio, who noted several profound abnormalities of the lung tissue. Not long after that, Darryl's breathing worsened and he was shipped to our ICU. And then he got the breathing tube and the ventilator.

I could see that Darryl's lip had been split open when the breathing tube was tunneled down his throat, and it reminded me of the lady from Mass General ER with the pet toucan. If it didn't heal properly, his scar might resemble Don's surgically repaired cleft palate. "I can also come back," I offered. "You must be exhausted."

An anesthesiologist once told our Harvard Medical School class that the ease of intubation was inversely related to neck flab; in the professor's opinion the most challenging patient in Boston would be the mayor, Thomas Menino. Based on his body type Darryl was undoubtedly difficult to intubate, and that's presumably why his lip had been split open. I glanced around his room, waiting for him to speak. There were no flowers, no get well cards; just a pile of XXXL clothes in a clear plastic bag. Where was his family? Was he someone, like Benny, who would pass the hospital days in solitude?

"Yeah," Darryl said softly, staring down at his abdomen. "I don't really want to talk. Don't want to talk to anyone."

"I understand."

"Just want to get out of here."

"Of course. We're gonna get you out of here as soon as it's safe."

"Cool. Hope it's soon."

"It will be." I decided to make one last go of it. I moved my head so that it more fully entered his field of vision. "I've been sick and alone before," I said. "And it sucked." I drew on my time taking the HIV medications. "I felt like I was gonna die and nobody cared." Darryl exhaled deeply; it was the largest breath I'd seen him take on his own. "But people do care. Everyone here cares about you." He remained silent, but I thought I saw a nod. I wanted to ask about his family, but I didn't want to risk opening a wound. "If you just let me ask you a few questions, I'll leave you alone. For the rest of the day. Just a few quick—"

"Fine."

"Okay," I said, turning to the questions I'd scribbled on my scut list. "Did you, out of curiosity, did you get the flu shot this year?"

"Nope."

"Why not?"

"Didn't think to."

"I'm sure you saw a doctor before you started college. Didn't he or she offer it to you?"

"Yeah, probably."

"Why didn't you get it?"

"I don't know, man."

I noted a small patch of hypopigmented skin at the angle of his jaw and jotted down *vitiligo?* on my scut list. "Do you know how important it is for someone like you to get a flu shot?"

He raised an eyebrow. "Someone like me?"

"Someone with asthma." I rolled my scut list up like an old newspaper. "Were you depressed?"

He shook his head. "No."

"I get depressed as shit in the winter."

His eyes shifted to the window. "Who doesn't?"

"Sucks."

We sat in silence for more than a minute. "I also feel like shit," he said, "in the summer. Feel like shit all the time." It was a difficult thing to hear, but I was encouraged that he was talking.

"You ever . . . I'm not saying you should or shouldn't, but . . . you ever talk to anyone about it?"

His jaw clenched. "Like a sociologist?"

"I don't know, anyone. A psychiatrist."

"No."

"When I get depressed," I said, "I don't want to talk to anyone. I want the world to leave me alone. I just want to turn it all off." I thought about the times I'd been depressed. I recalled how, in a fit of despair, I'd screamed at my HIV pill bottles after I'd vomited up what little dinner I could swallow. I thought about how much more difficult it all would've been if I had also been dealing with a chronic, debilitating illness. And if I'd been left to handle things on my own.

I tried to imagine Darryl's inner world, but I couldn't. His life was different from mine and he hadn't given me much to help me understand what he was going through or how I could help him. And I wasn't a mental health professional, so perhaps it wasn't my place to fully investigate these issues. I had learned this detail about the flu shot, and that was significant. Darryl rolled over in bed and yawned. "I'm good, man. Really. Kinda beat, actually. Just want to be left alone, honestly."

"Right," I said, looking at my pager. "Glad we got that tube out."

"Same."

"So . . . to be continued?"

"Sure."

I closed the tan curtain and headed back to the lounge.

"I think we have our answer," I said to Don a minute later. "He didn't get the flu shot." Don held a *New England Journal of Medicine* in his left hand and was typing with his right. Like many of my colleagues, Don set his password so that it could be typed with one hand, allowing orders to be entered at breakneck speed. "And he's depressed," I added, while taking a seat on the black leather couch.

"I'd be depressed, too," Don said.

"Really depressed."

"Any plan to act on it?"

"No interest in talking to a psychiatrist."

"That's not the question." He typed a final order and spun toward me. "There's an algorithm," he said. "If someone is depressed, the follow-up question is: Do you have homicidal or suicidal thoughts? If yes, do you have a plan to act on those thoughts?"

"Got it."

"There's a big difference between 'My roommate bums me out' and 'My roommate bums me out and I'm going to murder him next Tuesday with my new AK-47.'"

"Obviously."

Don tapped his index finger on the keyboard. "Suppose he does tell you that he has a plan. Plans to do something bad. Then what?"

"Call the cops, certainly." I hadn't yet met a patient who was actively planning to harm himself or someone else. I mostly thought of my patients as kind, temporarily debilitated beings in need of help, not deranged monsters capable of harming others.

"What about patient-doctor confidentiality, Matt? If a patient tells you about something devious in confidence—a plan to hurt someone or whatever—can you tell the cops?"

"I suppose I'd consult the hospital ethicist."

"That's passing the buck, Dr. McCarthy."

"I'd try to talk him out of it. That goes without saying."

"You haven't done your outpatient elective yet, have you?" Don asked.

"No."

"I take it you're not familiar with *Tarasoff*?" I shook my head. "One minute." He printed out a document and handed it to me. "Read this."

It was a summary of *Tarasoff v. Regents of the University of California*, a court case that all Columbia residents were eventually exposed to. In the summer of 1969, I read, as Don returned to his *New England Journal of Medicine*, a graduate student at Cal Berkeley told his psychologist that he was going to kill a woman, Tatiana Tarasoff, who had rejected his advances. The graduate student was briefly committed but ultimately set free. Several months later, he murdered Tarasoff by stabbing her to death. Neither Tarasoff nor her parents were ever given any warning about the threat and sued. The case went before the California Supreme Court, where it was ruled that a physician or mental health professional has a duty not only to a patient but also to individuals who are specifically being threatened by a patient. "The protective privilege ends," the majority opinion reads, "where the public peril begins."

"Well?" Don asked after I had put the paper down.

"I'm gonna talk to Darryl later today. See where his head is at. I don't think it's anything like that." I remembered that I'd promised him no more questions today.

Once again I marveled at all I was expected to master. Beyond the medical knowledge and procedures, beyond writing clear, informative notes and interacting with a wildly diverse hospital staff, I had to understand bioethics. I had to be familiar with court cases and legal precedents. I needed to know what to do in situations I'd never considered. The professional expectations were breathtaking.

"Told me his roommate calls him fat as fuck," Don said, still staring at the journal.

The words startled me. Don had already gotten Darryl to talk more than I had. How? My residents were always one step ahead of me. Or several. "I'll talk to him."

"Fine," Don said, "but don't do it now. We've got a lumbar puncture, two central lines, and a paracentesis that need to get done."

"Got it. I'll grab the stuff."

Three hours later, as I was finishing up the lumbar puncture, I caught Darryl Jenkins out of the corner of my eye. He was on a stretcher, wrapped in several blankets, with that plastic bag of clothes on his lap. His asthma had been stabilized and he no longer needed to be in the

ICU. He was being transferred to a general medicine floor and would probably be home in a matter of days.

But I hadn't gone back to talk to him. I had been too busy sticking needles in other patients. I needed to ask him if he'd ever thought of harming himself or another person, like his roommate. It felt like a small betrayal, like I was suggesting that I thought he was capable of something heinous. It just didn't seem right to ask Darryl—a kid who'd almost died because of an asthma exacerbation—if he thought about committing unspeakable acts because he was unhappy.

I dropped my pen and scut list and rushed over to his stretcher. "Hey," I said. "Congrats on getting out of here."

Darryl was staring into a cell phone and didn't look up. "Thanks, man."

This wasn't the moment to ask him about homicidal or suicidal thoughts, but someone needed to. Someone who was better trained than I was. I motioned to the patient escort to give us a minute. "Darryl," I said, leaning in close to his face, "can I ask something of you? It's nothing major."

He was texting and didn't look up. "Me do *you* a favor?"

"Yeah. But I want to run it by you first." I paused to consider my words. This was my final shot with him. "If we send in a mental health, um, if we send in a psychiatrist or whatever, will you speak with that person?"

He put down the phone and looked up at me. "Why?"

"Because I think it's important." As he stared me up and down, my pager went off. I quickly silenced it. "I can give you a longer explanation if you'd like, but the short answer is that I think you'd benefit from talking with someone about depression." He continued to stare, not saying a word. "So would I," I added. "I'd benefit from talking to someone, too."

He shrugged.

"It won't take long," I went on. "And I think it's important."

He received a text and picked up his phone. "Sure, man."

"Really?"

"Yeah, it's fine."

I hadn't expected him to agree so easily. My body had been mildly tensed for a longer bout of convincing, and now I wasn't sure what to do with the extra energy. I fought back a smile. It was a small victory—some might not even call it a victory, but I did. I considered it a tremendous victory.

Darryl might've been placating me—who knows what he'd even say to the psychiatrist?—but I had gotten him to let me create an opportunity for him to get better. And in some ways that was just as valuable as making him better myself. That, I realized, was the long game Jim O'Connell was playing with his patients, the kind I would need to play with people like Darryl and Dre. Their maladies were both immediate problems and symptoms of deeper problems. Convincing Darryl Jenkins to get a flu shot would be a start; it might save him for a year. Convincing him to care enough about himself to do it every year—that was the long-term goal. "Reaching" him, it seemed, might be as simple as pointing him on that path, hoping he'd eventually walk it himself.

"Terrific," I said. "We'll have someone come by later today."

Darryl looked over at the escort. "Just get me outta here."

We shook hands and I gave him a gentle nudge on the shoulder. "You got it."

A moment later, he was wheeled out of the unit and I never saw him again.

PART V

37

"It's freakin' ridiculous," Don said as he devoured the last slice of pepperoni pizza. It was mid-March, and more than six weeks had passed since that final exchange with Darryl Jenkins in the ICU. I'd just started a two-week stretch working nights on the general medicine service and had again been randomly paired with Don. He and I were outside of a patient's room on the sixth floor, standing before a large handwritten sign:

Male visitors must be announced

"Our new patient," Don said, tilting his head at the sign, "from Saudi Arabia. All sorts of nonsense."

Don shook his head while I was quietly reliving what now qualified as the wildest thing I'd seen in the hospital. A week earlier, during an arrest, a cardiothoracic surgeon had cracked a woman's chest open at the bedside and squeezed her heart. A room of stunned doctors and nurses had looked on in silence as the patient expired, and I'd had two nightmares about it. When it was over, our blood-splattered white coats had looked like a series of Jackson Pollock paintings. There had been an eerie silence as we gently filed out of the room, collectively dazed. Working nights was now a welcome relief—I didn't want to have that dream again. "What's up?" I asked.

"Just tried to examine her," Don said, "but the husband said I can't touch her. She's in a burka with just a tiny eye slit. He won't let her speak for herself. It's absurd."

I thought back to the cultural competency seminar and Marjorie, the student who would recuse herself from treating a Muslim. Would she really just throw up her hands and walk away? Was that what Don was about to do? It was odd seeing him so flustered. I fixated on the tomato sauce that had accumulated at the corners of his mouth.

"How am I supposed to make a diagnosis if I can't lay my hands on the patient?"

I shrugged; the master diagnostician had been stymied. "I'm not sure."

Behind the door was a young woman with a swollen, throbbing, ruby red knee. She'd been diagnosed with a tumor near the kneecap over New Year's, and it was our job to determine if her new fever was from the cancer, the treatment, or an infection. Don had every reason to be frustrated, but I wondered if he was making a tactical error by letting his emotions get involved. We needed to play the hand we were dealt.

"So what do we do?" I asked.

"What do *you* suggest we do, Dr. McCarthy? I will defer to you." Don had gradually been giving me this kind of latitude as we worked through patients. It was a way of pulling back the process and making me, and my fellow interns, more comfortable making decisions. I imagined myself walking a new intern through these scenarios, perhaps as a stall tactic while I gathered my own thoughts. "Take me through your thought process," he said, running his hands through his floppy hair. "I want to know how you think."

"Well, I suppose one option is to assume she has an infection and treat her. Give her broad antibiotics. Vancomycin and Zosyn. We haven't identified what might be causing the infection, but those two antibiotics would cover most bacteria."

"Okay."

"Another option is to get an MRI and hope that gives us the answer. Progression of the tumor or a new infection."

"Sure."

"But the test is expensive and perhaps unnecessary."

"Right."

"Or we could get another set of blood tests to see if her white blood cell count is rising."

"Certainly."

I folded my arms. "Or we tell the husband to get out of the way so we can actually examine the woman."

"And then get fired."

"I doubt that would happen."

"Fine. All of those suggestions are reasonable. But what would you actually do if I weren't here? What's your move, Doctor?"

I imagined the unknowable woman under the burka and hedged. "I would get an MRI."

"Then that's what we'll do."

We walked over to a set of computers and he put in the MRI order. "Is that . . . is that what you would've done?" I asked as I polished off my Gatorade. "The MRI?"

"No."

We stared at each other in silence. Then Don looked at his watch and informed me that I was free to take a twenty-minute nap.

"I'm not wrong," I said defensively.

"I didn't say that you were."

Moments later, I crawled into a call room bed and thought about what had just transpired. I was comfortable with the choice I had made. I had treated hundreds of patients and was reaching the point where I could reasonably disagree with my superior and not feel bad about it.

I saw doctors disagree all the time. Ours was merely a difference of opinion, two contrasting ways of trying to answer a question that had no obvious answer. A few months earlier, I would have fretted on it for days. This felt like a snapshot moment—one that let me see how much the passage of time had changed me as a doctor.

Before long I drifted off to sleep. Soon my mind had transported me to a beach, far, far away from the hospital. Then I heard a knock at the door.

"Can't sleep," Don said.

I had been in a deep slumber, dead to the world, about to order a cocktail with an umbrella in it. "Me either."

"Hypothetical," he said, crawling onto the top bunk. "Ready?" He was clearly still worked up about the woman with the red knee, but he needed something else to think about.

"You know I love these."

"Okay," he said, "they're saying flu season might be bad this year, that we might have to ration ventilators if New York gets hit hard."

"Sure."

"We're down to our last ventilator in the ICU and two patients need it: a thirty-two-year-old pregnant woman and a six-year-old boy. Who you gonna give it to?"

I took out my notebook, continuing to add to my list of hypotheticals. I planned to use them on next year's crop of interns. "No other options. I have to pick one?"

"Yes."

"Which one is more sick?"

"They are both equally sick. Without the ventilator they will each perish in minutes. With it, they'll each live a happy, healthy life on Martha's Vineyard."

"The Vineyard can be dreary in the winter."

"That's the scenario. You're stalling."

"Reflexively I'd pick the mother," I said. "Save two lives. Wait . . . how far along in the pregnancy?"

"Four months. She can't deliver the baby." He sounded surprised. "If I take the baby out of it, would you save the kid?"

These exchanges helped us prepare for unexpected clinical scenarios, but they also helped us get to know each other; it was fascinating to discover how differently colleagues could approach the same ethical quagmire. In this case, however, the answer seemed obvious. "Yes," I said. "Remove pregnancy from the equation and I'd save the six-year-old before the thirty-two-year-old."

"Where do you stand on abortion? Pro-choice?"

"Um . . . why?"

"Just curious when you think life begins. You're not a life-begins-at-conception guy, I take it?"

"Even if I don't consider the unborn child a viable being, I'd save the pregnant mother."

"Huh, I'd pick the kid."

"What? Why?"

"I couldn't do that to a kid, Matt. I couldn't."

"What if the mother was pregnant with twins?"

He leaned his head over the edge of the bed. "You just opened a whole other can of worms, my friend. In that case I'd pick the mother."

Neither of us could know that a swine flu pandemic was mere weeks away and that we would be called to very real emergency meetings dealing with the possible issue of ventilator rationing. Some of the most contentious arguments I witnessed as an intern dealt with the hypothetical methods for allocating resources in the face of uncertainty. Those clashes about ventilators—which occasionally bubbled over into shouting matches—invariably drew me back to Benny, who was still languishing because of the UNOS organ-sharing algorithm. When you're advocating for your patient, you don't care about the wisdom of a construct that benefits someone who is not your patient.

"Okay, I've got one," I said. "Guy spends a year living in the CCU waiting for an organ transplant that never arrives. How much is his hospital bill?"

"That's not"—Don, still peering over the edge of the bed, trailed off and contorted his face like he was staring into a bright light— "really a hypothetical."

Like nearly all of my colleagues, Don had taken care of Benny during the last year, but I couldn't tell if Benny's saga had affected him (or anyone else, for that matter) the way it had me. "I suppose it's not."

"Probably a million bucks," Don said. "Maybe two. With all the nursing costs and food and specialists, it's probably closer to two." He shook his head. "It's kinda mind-boggling."

Mind-boggling was an understatement. A slew of more appropriate adjectives came to mind: *incredible, outrageous, ridiculous.* And who was paying for it all? His insurance company? Taxpayers? I never asked him; I didn't want to know. "You think he's getting that heart?" I asked.

Benny's fate had truly become an obsession with me. I now saw so much of the healthcare system—particularly the inefficiency and the excess—through the lens of his situation. Was it really that bad to order an extraneous test or two when millions were being spent on just one guy? Did it really matter if someone's discharge was held up by a single day when he'd been held hostage for months?

"Honestly?" Don asked. "No, Matt, I don't think he's getting the heart."

I shook my head and picked up an EKG book. "I'd like to disagree with you. But I'm not sure I can."

"I think one of these times," Don went on, "he's gonna need to be intubated and something happens, maybe it takes too long, maybe the tube goes in the wrong spot, and he's gonna have a cardiac arrest and that'll be it."

The thought made me shudder. Who would tell his family? Who would run the cardiac arrest? I hoped it would be Baio.

"You're bumming me out," Don said, returning to his pillow. "Okay, I got another. Would you rather marry Madonna or an adult film actress?"

I was happy to change the subject. "Porn star?"

"Yes."

"Madonna now or—"

"Yeah," he said, "now."

"Is the porn star still, ah, active in the industry?"

"Yes."

"And is she performing to pay off my loans or because she loves the work?"

"Loves the work."

"And what phase is Madonna in?"

"Chiseled cougar in need of a boy toy."

"Has the porn star ever won any awards for her work?"

"Several."

I wondered if Lalitha and Ariel and Meghan talked about this kind of nonsense with their supervising residents. I knew they talked about silly stuff with me, but I was curious if it extended beyond our pod. Were other doctors in other call rooms trying to make each other laugh? "This is a tough one," I said. "I imagine holidays would be difficult with the porn star. How does my mother feel about the starlet?"

"At your wedding she wrestled the microphone away from the emcee and said, 'I can't believe my son is marrying a fucking porn star.'"

"Yikes."

"Otherwise, the relationship has been cordial."

"Where do we live?"

"Scottsdale, Arizona."

"Naturally. How do my friends feel about the porn gal?"

"Friends from college think she's really cool. Friends from med school do not."

"And does Madonna treat me as her intellectual equal?"

"No."

"Am I allowed to make eye contact with her?"

"Madonna allows you to look directly at her three times a day."

"My sister would be pumped if—"

"Your sister thinks you're gay."

I took a deep breath. "I think I gotta go with Madonna."

He rubbed my shoulder and fought off a smile. "Dr. McCarthy, I have posed that hypothetical to perhaps a dozen interns this year and no one, no one, has taken that long to conclude that Madonna is the preferable life partner."

38

The following night, Don and I were in the emergency room examining a woman transferred to Columbia from a nursing home when I saw Sam out of the corner of my eye. I removed the stethoscope from the woman's chest and headed toward my patient. As I strode across the room, I felt my phone buzz. It was a text from Heather: BOTTLE OF WINE WAITING FOR YOU AT HOME.

The words made me smile. I had spent the year learning to take care of patients, and she'd largely spent the year taking care of me. Heather had acknowledged that seeing me unwell for so long had taken a toll on her; it had been difficult living with a humorless zombie, someone wholly focused on trying to avoid a mental or physical breakdown. CAN'T WAIT, I wrote back.

Heather possessed an innate sense of when I needed reassurance and when I just needed to get drunk. Or laugh. And now that I was off the HIV meds, I could finally do both. Regaining a feeling of normalcy in my private life, I discovered, helped me to cope with the emotional roller coaster of being a doctor. I could recharge at home, just as Ashley had once instructed. It was fun getting to see the real me again, Heather said, and I felt the same way.

Now that the needle stick episode was behind us, we began to speak more openly about just how awful that period had been. Heather confessed that she had responded internally with dark humor, telling herself that if I did get AIDS, we'd make lemonAIDS. I'm not sure if that line would've made me laugh or cry when I was living with the uncertainty of my diagnosis. Probably both. But the fact that she could now tell me these things helped me appreciate just how far we'd come. I put the phone away and greeted my patient.

"Sam," I said, "what are you doing here?" He was lying on a stretcher, flashing those champagne-colored teeth around the emergency room. It was strange to see him outside of my primary care clinic.

"Dr. McCarthy," he said, extending a callused hand, "it seems I've gotten myself in a bit of a pickle."

I grabbed a chair. "Talk to me."

"Started having chest pains again so I called your office. But it was closed so I came here." Over the past few months we'd grown closer—detecting Sam's subtle heart murmur in a routine clinic visit had been a turning point in our initially awkward relationship—but I'd watched in vain as his health steadily deteriorated. The long list of problems that had flashed on my screen before his first visit had proven to be accurate, and I'd been seeing him on a monthly basis in my clinic, sometimes overbooking him, but it wasn't enough. Because of my hectic hospital schedule, I was only in the primary clinic one afternoon per week, and it left me with the constant, gnawing sensation that I wasn't sufficiently there for him. "They did some blood work," he said, "EKG, the usual stuff. Gotta say I appreciate you coming in to see me at, what, two in the morning."

Did he need to know I was working nights and our rendezvous was merely a coincidence? I squeezed his hand. "You're gonna get through this." It was something I said to nearly all of my hospitalized patients, and it was a remark that I regularly wrestled with. In some cases—in a great many cases, really—I didn't mean it. I tried to remain vague, never saying exactly what the person was going to pull through, but I knew when the odds were tragically stacked against a patient. Still, I felt the need to be positive, to offer hope to someone who'd been given up on. So I told people they were going to pull through something that maybe they weren't, and I wasn't sure if that was wrong.

"I know," Sam said. "I know."

"Where are things now?"

"They say I'm having a heart attack. A light heart attack."

A light heart attack. What a weird term. "You look damn good for having a heart attack. Even a light one."

"They say I need a cardiac catheterization."

I couldn't hear that term without thinking of Gladstone or Denise Lundquist. So much had changed since those first days in the cardiac care unit—I occasionally cringed at my initial incompetence—but in other ways, very little was different. I still thought about Professor Gladstone and Ms. Lundquist like they were my patients. I vividly recalled the tactile sensation of examining their lymph nodes, of pressing my stethoscope against their skin, of retracting an eyelid to peer into a pupil. "Okay," I said, glancing at Sam's vital signs. "It's a fairly minor procedure. You'll get through it."

"But the dye they have to use might screw up my kidneys."

"Right."

"The cardiologist says I might need preemptive dialysis. But the kidney doc tells me that won't do any good and is refusing to do dialysis. So, here I am."

"Here you are."

Moranis had warned me that this day was coming; Sam's heart and kidneys were on a collision course, and we agreed the kidneys would have to be sacrificed. Sam and I had discussed this extensively over the past few months, and although I wasn't a kidney or heart specialist, he knew I was his advocate.

To fully explore the anatomy of Sam's injured heart, the cardiologists would need to inject a special dye into him. But that dye was known to harm the kidneys, and the nephrologists warned that his already damaged organs couldn't handle the insult. Injecting the dye could destroy his kidneys and force him to go on dialysis. He'd need to visit a dialysis center three times per week for a long time—possibly the rest of his life—and might lose the ability to urinate on his own.

If that happened, the cardiologists might get in trouble—the need for dialysis after cardiac catheterization was a reportable offense—so there was talk of starting dialysis prior to injecting the dye. But the data supporting such a maneuver was sparse, and the nephrologists weren't interested in doing it. So we were at a crossroads, one that left me utterly perplexed. Moranis told me that if anyone suggested there was an easy answer for Sam, they didn't appreciate the complexity of his situation.

"Stuck in the middle," I said, fingering the loose flesh on my neck. "This is a tough one." I imagined Sam's heart and kidneys in a boxing ring, fighting it out as Axel's words once again wafted into my head: *Do not fuck with the pancreas.* "You shoulda called me," I added, "directly."

Because my hours in the primary care clinic were so limited, Sam was in the habit of texting me when he got his blood pressure checked at the grocery store. Moranis had warned against doling out my cell phone number to patients, but it was the only way to keep tabs on everyone. I thought about Jim O'Connell and what he did for his patients, wading out into the night, searching for life, searching for illness. Giving out my phone number seemed like the least I could do. I had spent so much of the year trying to connect with patients, but when I gave Sam and others my personal number, they were able to feel a connection with me. "I'm serious," I added.

"Any chance," Sam said, "any chance you guys can put your heads together and sort this one out?"

"I'll see what I can do."

"Thank you," he said, putting a hand on his chest. "I'll just hang here, having a heart attack."

I walked across the emergency room and returned to Don. "Got a hypothetical for you," I said. "My clinic patient over there is having a heart attack. Needs a cath but no one wants to touch him. Cardiology's afraid they'll destroy his kidneys, and the nephrologists don't want to dialyze him preemptively. What do we do?"

Don stared at my chest. "Again, not a hypothetical if it's actually happening."

"What do you think?"

"It's a tough one."

"Right? I can see both sides."

We looked at Sam, who was now reading *The New Yorker*. It must have been an exceedingly light heart attack, I thought. "Remember," Don said, "you're not the first to encounter whatever situation is stumping you. Never forget that."

"Good point."

"Could mention it to Dave," he said, pointing at our chief resident, who was moonlighting in the ER to make a few extra bucks. I hadn't had a one-on-one meeting since that encounter in his office, the one where he expressed concern that five interns were leaving our program and I admitted I was struggling. It had been an uncomfortable interaction—I had replayed the dialogue in my head dozens of times—and I was left with the impression that Dave was trying to make my life more difficult. That belief may have been misguided, but it was how I felt, and even the improvement of my station at the hospital in subsequent months hadn't quite dislodged the feeling.

I also wasn't excited to venture over to Dave's section of the emergency room, Area B, which held a large pit of dangerously inebriated or psychotic men and women. These erratic patients were monitored by a half dozen improbably large security guards, and in my brief experience, it was nearly impossible to set foot in Area B without having some sort of bodily fluid flung at you.

"Dave," I called out as I approached the pit. "Hey."

"Big guy!" he said, sticking out a hand. "How are things?"

"Fine. Quick question."

He curtsied. "How may I be of service?"

It wasn't clear if chief residents were the select few who truly retained the pseudoenthusiasm of intern year or were simply the best at faking being fake. "I got a bit of a situation." I quickly recounted Sam's scenario and asked for Dave's advice.

"Let's set up a talk!" Dave said. "We'll get a cardiologist and a nephrologist to come and duke it out." He pretended my belly was a punching bag and threw a few light taps to my midsection. It was weird. "It'll be great, Matt!" He typed a few words into his phone and smiled.

"But, Dave, what do we do now? Like, right now."

"Let's talk it out," he said, putting an arm around me. "Introduce me to Sam."

I still didn't know what to make of Dave. I couldn't say why, but he rubbed me the wrong way. Like he'd sell me out if we were both suspected of a crime or squash me if it meant professional advancement. But why? He hadn't really done anything to me. Maybe he had just been worried I was going to leave medicine. What if I was a bad judge of character? What if Dave was one of the guys in my corner and I didn't realize it?

I stared intently at him, hoping his facial expression would tip me off. Was this guy on my team? As I glared at his thin lips, I wondered how often I had rubbed people the wrong way—and not just doctors but patients. How often did they find my probing questions too much? How frequently did my attempts to connect with people backfire?

Dave and I walked toward the other end of the ER, and I pointed out Sam. He looked calm, almost like he was on vacation and the stretcher was a chaise lounge.

"Hard to believe," Dave said, "that a new crop of interns will be taking your place soon. You ready to have your own intern to boss around?"

"Ha. What do you think?"

"I think you've come a long way from those mopey days . . . after the needle stick."

"Mopey?"

"I kid, I kid. I think you're doing great." My index finger still had the occasional phantom pain where I'd jabbed myself, but I appreciated the compliment. Dave always caught me off guard. "I've seen your faculty evaluations, Matt. Really strong. I was actually wondering," he said, "if you'd be a tour guide for the new interns. And for next year's applicants. We think you'd be perfect."

We? I fought off a grin. "I'd be delighted."

At some point I had apparently quantum-leapt into the body of a reasonably competent, capable doctor. I could feel it was true, but couldn't quite figure out when it had happened. When had I gone from *we're worried you're decompensating* to *wanna be a tour guide*? Where was that transformative scene, like Don's master diagnosis? Maybe it was something more gradual, like demonstrating that I could consistently function on eight minutes of sleep or that I could navigate a needle under duress. Perhaps, like Don, I had cemented my reputation with just one patient—but who?

"Awesome," Dave said, "just give people a sense of what it's actually like to work here."

I looked over at the pit of dangerous patients in Area B and smiled. "Sure."

My mind began to wander, as it often did late at night. Could I accurately represent the diorama of hospital life at Columbia? Or the strange enchantments of practicing medicine? Could I explain how wonderfully insane it all is? I thought back to the first few weeks with Baio in the CCU; did the tribulations of intern year appear different now than they had in July? I didn't think so, but I couldn't be certain. "So," I said, transitioning out of my neurotic inner monologue, "my patient Sam. Let me give you the full story."

39

Walking out of the ED hours later, after further testing revealed that Sam wasn't having a heart attack—not even a light one—I saw another old friend sitting alone in the waiting room. "Dre?" I whispered to myself.

She had put on some weight—at least twenty pounds, maybe more—but there was no mistaking her. She was wearing a bright green sundress, large sunglasses, and slippers; it was probably forty degrees outside, but she was dressed for summer. "Dre?" I said, somewhat louder. So much had happened since she'd walked out on me, and I still had many questions. She still had those bumps on her face, but they were smaller and there were fewer of them.

Rarely is a physician able to pinpoint someone who leaves such a lasting impression, but she, like Benny, was one of them for me. "Hey," I said, taking a seat next to her, "it's Dr. McCarthy." She didn't respond. Perhaps Dre was a pseudonym she'd made up on the spot and didn't remember using. "I was your doctor a few months ago."

Seeing her allowed a tangle of buried thoughts to emerge. I remembered how much I'd felt like a failure when she vanished. I was just another person in her life who didn't get it, another stiff in a white coat who wasn't worth her time. Part of the process of rebuilding my confidence in the months that followed had entailed learning how to avoid taking failures personally. But like a first love lost, Dre's departure still stung. It was hard to be rational about it, even in retrospect. What had I done wrong? I still desperately wanted to know.

After her middle-of-the-night departure, I did some digging and dis-covered that Eminem and Dr. Dre had done a duet called "Forgot About Dre." I'd occasionally played it when I took my HIV pills and had the lyrics tucked away for a moment such as this. I knew she was battling several chronic illnesses and would inevitably pop up in our emergency room again. But I didn't expect it to be now, just before dawn on a chilly night in March. Her eyes were closed, so I gave her a gentle nudge. She looked better—not great—and the added weight suited her well. Did she remember me? I quietly said the lyrics in her direction:

"Everybody wanna talk like they got somethin' to say . . ." I scanned the room; no one was watching us. "But nothin' comes out when they move their lips just a bunch of gibberish."

Dre flinched and her jaw went slack; it was a preposterous thing to say to a patient, but it's what I said.

"Em?" Her frown gave way to a wide-ranging smile.

"In the flesh," I said. She *did* remember.

"No shit."

"Indeed." I gave her a once-over. "You doing okay?"

"Yeah, yeah. Just need a checkup."

"In the ER?"

She didn't respond.

"Well," I said, "you look good." I lightly touched the fabric of her dress as she tapped a matching handbag at her feet, and she whispered, "Calfskin."

I thought back to that agonizing moment when I'd discovered she had vanished. "So, where in the world did you go that night?" I asked. "The last time I saw you. Why did you leave the hospital? How did—"

"Long story, Em."

"I got time." My pager vibrated as I spoke. Don was summoning me to see a young man with priapism—that dreaded scenario where an erection lasts more than four hours. It is an excruciating condition, one that on occasion necessitates an injection directly into the penis to prevent dangerous blood clots. I had a minute with Dre, maybe less.

"I just want to know," I said, "why you chose to—"

"Em, you a real doctor?"

"Yes, of course."

She grinned. "Just checkin'."

"Please tell me you're taking the . . . the meds. All of them."

"I am!" She extended an arm and squeezed my shoulder. "Started seeing Dr. Chanel. She hooks me up."

"Wonderful." She felt my other shoulder and gave it a squeeze. "You're bigger than I remember, Em."

We both had put on a bit of weight. "You wanna hear something funny?" I asked. "In med school, one of my instructors told me my physicality was intimidating to other students."

"Physicality?"

"Yeah."

"Who uses that word?"

"Weird, right?"

She held up her hand and counted out the syllables. "Phys-i-cal-i-ty."

"So honestly, Dre, where did you go that night?"

"Out."

"I know this is kind of a weird thing to say, but I was really hurt. Seriously."

She touched my leg. "I'm taking the pills. But I had to go. I had to. I'm sorry." Many of my poorer patients temporarily disappeared on the first or fifteenth of the month to collect unemployment or disability, but they usually came back the same day. It wasn't an ideal situation, but my hands were generally tied. "Chanel hooked me up," she added. "I'm good."

"Well, you look good."

She touched my face, like she had in the hospital. "So do you."

"One more thing," I said, quickly scanning another text on my pager. "Did you start taking the pills because of . . . because of me? Because of the conversations we had?"

"Honestly?"

"Yes, honestly." I closed my eyes. I never willed my patients to answer questions the way I wanted them to, but I was now.

"Oh, Em."

"Be straight with me." Or just humor me.

Dre turned her head slightly. "Honestly, no." She stood up, straightened her dress, and patted me on the leg. "I've got to go. Good-bye, Em."

PART VI

40

After my two-week stint of nights with Don—he and I had exhausted hundreds of hypotheticals during our fortnight together—I was shipped uptown to work a monthlong rotation in the intensive care unit of the Allen Hospital. Located near the northern tip of Manhattan, the Allen was a three-hundred-bed community hospital on 220th Street where Columbia interns spent one month learning the art of geriatric medicine and a separate month running the intensive care unit. The structure of supervision was a bit different uptown because in contrast to the Columbia behemoth on 168th Street—a topflight international referral center—patients at the modest, three-story Allen Hospital tended to have less acute, less complex medical conditions. And for that, we were all thankful.

At first blush, the assignment seemed somewhat contradictory. If patients at the Allen weren't that sick, why have an ICU? On an interminable northbound subway ride to 220th Street in early April, I wondered if, like Sam's allegedly light heart attack, I was about to begin work in a light intensive care unit. As the subway approached the hospital I considered how odd it was to think of humans in this way—as medically simple or complex, the chronically ill or the worried well—rather than as funny or kind or annoying. I was struck by how differently my mind worked now than it did just a few years ago. When did I begin to identify people first on the basis of physiology rather than personality? When did that accountant I was caring for become Salmonella Lady or Diarrhea Guy?

After ten months of being an intern, I no longer experienced life like a normal person. I couldn't watch a movie or read a magazine without drifting off to the hospital—to a procedure or an ambiguous diagnosis or a patient encounter—to relive the moment again and again, until something shook me out of the moment. I now found it hard to have a conversation without mentioning something I had seen or done at work. Ordering lunch at a deli, I'd be thinking about the patient who claimed he sat on a jar of Grey Poupon. Checking out at a grocery store, I'd be thinking about the lung blebs.

I now viewed everything through the lens of medicine. It wasn't something I had planned or particularly wanted, it just happened. When I saw someone on the street with a limp, I now fixated on how it might have happened—stroke? fractured bone? muscle-wasting disease?—until I felt confident in my armchair diagnosis. I found myself staring at oddly shaped moles on the subway and at low-set ears in the park. What caused these things? I couldn't let it go until I'd formulated some sort of hypothesis.

I desperately wanted to become a superb doctor, but as the year wore on I also found myself wanting to remember what it was like to not be a physician—to just be a guy going for a stroll with an uncluttered mind and an armful of groceries. A guy who didn't act quickly and decisively, someone who could make eye contact without thinking about ophthalmology. I wanted to be a doctor *and* a normal person. Was that possible? Or were the two mutually exclusive? I hoped I would never have to choose, but in some ways it felt like I already had.

When I stepped into the Allen ICU for that first thirty-hour shift in April, I discovered that my pod would be supervised by just one third-year resident (rather than four second-year residents) and that this resident would be supervised by two attending physicians. This had presumably been explained to me months earlier, during orientation, when intern year had been laid out in a series of presentations, but I had forgotten the details. I had become remarkably nearsighted over the course of the year, focused on what I needed to know to get through the day, rather than what might take place in the weeks and months ahead.

The entire Allen ICU team was to go home at 8:00 P.M., meaning I was left to hold down the fort on my own overnight. I would have backup, of course, in the form of an overnight attending physician who was admitting his or her own patients in another part of the hospital. But once the sun went down, I was essentially alone.

If scheduled toward the end of the academic year, the Allen ICU was said to be the ideal setting for a promising intern to become comfortable making tough decisions in solitude, without the second-guessing and hand-holding of a more senior resident. But it was also a place where mistakes would be amplified; making the wrong diagnosis or selecting an improper medication could inflict real harm rather than just a tongue-lashing from a supervisor. I had heard stories of interns breaking down in tears from the existential terror of presiding over an ICU in solitude. As the sun settled below the Hudson River and I said good-bye to my ICU colleagues on that first night alone, I only had one thought: *Don't fuck up.*

Glancing around the ICU—the room was about the size of a Little League infield—I noticed the fluorescent lights weren't as bright as they were at Columbia and the place smelled different, vaguely antiseptic, as if the tiled floor had just been mopped with chlorine and the room had been infused with industrial-strength air freshener. It wasn't better or worse than the hospital on 168th Street, just different, like I had moved into a new apartment—a strange sublet with unfamiliar neighbors and appliances that I'd eventually get used to but for now felt foreign.

Before me in the unit were a dozen unconscious bodies attached to ventilators and large-bore IVs, just like at Columbia. There were bleating blood pressure monitors, energetic nurses, and grieving families, just like at Columbia. There were familiar stacks of EKGs and day-old bagels, but there was no Baio and there was no Don. It was just me, alone with a group of very sick, very complicated patients. This was not ICU Lite.

I stared at my scut list on that first evening alone and tried to devise a plan of attack. Where would Baio begin? How would Ashley triage this list? There were perhaps two dozen assignments that needed to be completed before sunrise, and I could do them in any order I wanted. I'd be able to do them with ease if the night remained uneventful, but it would be foolish to assume the night would be quiet. Unforeseen developments—fibrillating hearts, profound electrolyte disturbances, intractable vomiting—would undoubtedly keep me busy, not to mention new patients coming up from the ED. I slung my stethoscope around my neck, checked my pager, and made my way to the nearest patient.

The small room was dark and cool, shielded from the ICU's fluorescent lighting by a large beige curtain that ran around the perimeter. An LCD screen that projected ventilator settings faintly illuminated the mottled skin of a chemically sedated, morbidly obese Vietnamese woman with pneumonia and impossibly long fingernails. As I approached the bed, I felt a silent partner at my side. First it was the voice of Ashley, gently reminding me to feel for hidden lymph nodes; then it was Jim O'Connell, reminding me to peek under the fingernails. I introduced myself to this unconscious woman as a formality, knowing she would be unable to respond. But I spoke loudly, just in case a word or phrase might register.

I felt ready for this challenge, but in those first solitary moments at the Allen, I realized how much I relied on others, how often I tugged the sleeve of a colleague and said, "Hey, quick question." For me, bouncing ideas and treatment plans off of others had become a way of life, a safeguard to prevent a medical mishap. But now, I didn't have that option. I put on a disposable gown and a pair of gloves and lightly pressed my stethoscope to the woman's sweltering chest.

Soon Don was in my head, forcing me to describe the sound of the woman's heart murmur in greater and greater detail. Glancing at her ample belly, I could hear him reminding me of the proper way to perform an abdominal exam. *Look, listen, palpate.* As I scribbled my findings and the voices bounced around my brain, I felt less alone. I knew that if my judgment failed me, memory would not. I had diagnosed and treated pneumonia so many times that I just needed to draw on prior experience to guide me.

During our series of nights together, Don and I had encountered pneumonia at least a dozen times, and with each successive case he had pulled back, giving me more authority to generate the differential diagnosis, order tests, and concoct a treatment plan. I had felt in control, and developed a modicum of comfort making important decisions, although I knew he was my safety net, double-checking my work in the background. And when Don disagreed with me, I no longer felt compelled to say, "I'm not wrong," even though I might have been. If I had made a real error, I knew he would've caught it.

"Continue broad-spectrum antibiotics for another twenty-four hours," I said softly, as I exited the Vietnamese woman's room, "and try to get her off the ventilator tomorrow." I briefly closed my eyes and imagined my erstwhile supervisors gently nodding in agreement. Then I scribbled the plan onto my scut list.

Moving on to the next patient—a frail Italian man with what had been dubbed a fever of unknown origin—I imagined the voice of Lalitha rattling off the uncommon causes of fever. *Don't forget about familial Mediterranean fever, Matty.* Then it was Ariel chiming in, reminding me of the more common causes of fever that might have been missed. *Did you check for tuberculosis, Dr. McCarthy?* So much of my medical knowledge had come from rounds, simply listening as my pod mates dissected hundreds and hundreds of cases. As I quickly jotted down vital signs, I felt the urge to text them: *Wish me luck!* or *Feel free to come back if you're bored at home!*

But I didn't text them. In fact, I took my cell phone out of my back pocket and placed it in the center of the unit, next to a computer keyboard. Service was so spotty in the hospital that doctors rarely communicated via cell phone; the thing would only serve as a distraction, and I wanted to immerse myself in the essence of being alone and unassisted. I knew it would take complete focus to get through the night without making a mistake.

I had seen and done so much since the Gladstone episode, and the pitiful note I'd written for Baio that had so enraged Sothscott. I was always someone who liked a challenge, but the Gladstone incident had transiently suppressed that, turning me into a gun-shy physician who was afraid of screwing up. Now I had finally moved beyond that, receiving enough positive feedback from supervising physicians—for my ability both to perform procedures and to present complex cases concisely during rounds—that being in charge of delivering care was no longer a stomach-churning thought. Now I could look at a patient like Carl Gladstone with unequal pupils and make a long list of things that could be responsible. I could narrow and rearrange that list, creating a hierarchy of probable causes, and from there I could page an expert—a neurologist, neurosurgeon, or ophthalmologist—to confirm or disprove my suspicions. I felt different now because I was different. After nearly a year of being an intern, I knew I was almost a real doctor. *Almost.*

After examining the remainder of the patients in the Allen ICU—there were no medical emergencies, just a handful of conversations with distraught, confused family members—another voice drifted into my head. *When you can eat, eat.* As I wandered over to a box of chocolate donuts in the center of the unit, the ward clerk handed me a telephone and said, "It's the emergency room." Here we go.

An ER physician named Dr. Brickow quickly introduced himself.

"Just examined a twenty-five-year-old guy named Dan Masterson," he said. "Guy's in rough shape, gonna need an ICU. I take it you have beds?"

I remembered the back-and-forth between Baio and Don, trying to find an ICU bed for Benny, as I scarfed down a donut. "We do." Masterson would be the first new patient I cared for alone. That responsibility no longer felt like a burden; it was something I wanted. "What's his deal?" I asked.

"It's a weird story," Brickow went on. "Wife gets pregnant with their second kid, so he switches jobs to pay the bills. Had to get a health clearance to start work and out of nowhere he tests positive for hep C."

I grabbed a plastic chair and took a seat. "Huh."

"Happened a few months ago."

"So what happened? Why's he here?" I started to create an illness narrative for this new patient. It was something I had learned from Don. It was his way of transforming a two-dimensional story about a set of discrete symptoms into a three-dimensional image of a human being grappling with a disease. It was often helpful, but it occasionally led me to jump to premature, unfounded conclusions.

The narrative started to come together in my mind: I imagined Dan Masterson's unkempt body stumbling into the Allen emergency room with belly pain. Or cirrhosis. He had prematurely aged—Dan was probably a young old man—and he'd initially chalked up his symptoms to stress. Trouble at work, having another kid, something like that. He'd ignored some warning signs—weight loss, shortness of breath—and now he was with us, clinging to life. I wondered if he was frail. I wondered what he was wearing. I wanted to know when he had contracted the virus and how his wife had reacted.

I took a sip from a can of soda and glanced around for a Styrofoam cup, wondering if I might need it for later. How sick was this guy? And would I know what to do? Suddenly, I wasn't feeling so eager to get a new patient. I hoped I wouldn't see a new medical condition tonight. I wanted something routine, something I could handle. I wasn't looking for a teachable moment, especially since there was no one around to teach me.

"Here's the strange part," Dr. Brickow said, the pitch of his voice rising slightly. "The guy walks in here from work a few hours ago—walking, talking, totally normal guy—and tells me he thinks he's gonna die."

I again recalled the terror I had experienced after the needle stick. I had felt that way more than a few times and I hadn't been *that* sick. "Yeah."

"And he tells me he's been doing some experimental treatment. Inhaled nitric oxide therapy."

"Really?"

"Yep. Found it on the Internet. Read some testimonials that it cures hep C, so he thought he'd give it a whirl."

I shook my head. "That's kinda weird." Earlier in the year, I had learned a bit about inhaled nitric oxide therapy after a patient in my clinic with sickle cell disease asked about it. It turned out there was a black market for the stuff and people were trying it for all sorts of diseases. But it wasn't a treatment for hep C.

Dr. Brickow covered his mouthpiece and gave an order to someone in the ER. Something about a CAT scan.

"So," I said, "I assume his wife knows he's—"

"That's the other thing . . . says he hasn't told his wife anything. And the second kid just arrived a month ago."

"Oh."

"Yeah, and I gotta warn you, he's going south quickly. Blood pressure is tanking. Probably need to tube him. I don't know if it's the nitric oxide or what."

"All right," I said, "send him on up. I'm ready." It was the only acceptable response, but I was fighting nerves. This scenario was a blank area on my canvas.

A few minutes later, the ICU doors burst open and a team of emergency room physicians and nurses wheeled Dan Masterson into the last open bed in the unit. Unlike Columbia's ICU, there was no unlucky corner pocket at the Allen. Frantic energy filled the room. "Lost the pulse," someone shouted as I scrambled over. "Start chest compressions," said another. My new admission, my first new patient, had flatlined en route to the ICU.

I quickly scooted up to the head of the stretcher and crashed into Dan Masterson's sternum with the heels of my hands. Before I'd even seen his face, before I'd noted what color hair or eyes he had, I had cracked one of his ribs. Probably two. I pumped up and down on his broken chest as another physician barked out orders, and in the midst of the madness—as a breathing tube was quickly snaked down his trachea and a nurse pumped adrenaline into his lifeless body—I stole a quick glance at my new patient. Dan Masterson looked nothing like what I had imagined. The man was large—well over six feet tall—and he had a barrel chest and thick, muscular arms. He had short blond hair, stormy green eyes, and tattoos all over his chest and abdomen. He looked like a youngish, healthy guy, not someone we should be trying to pull back from the brink of death.

A tall, slender ER physician stood at the foot of the stretcher, calmly leading the resuscitation as I furiously mashed on Masterson's chest. "I need calcium, insulin, and bicarb," the doctor said to the nurse next to him. Addressing the rest of us, he said, "The patient has been asystolic for three minutes. Please continue CPR."

Sweat accumulated on my forehead as I smashed my hands into Dan Masterson's sunken, lopsided chest. A few drops trickled off the tip of my nose and hit him in the neck. Soon the drops were landing on his face. After five minutes of compressions, my scrub top was drenched. As the minutes ticked by, I found myself smashing harder and harder on the lifeless body, searching in vain for a flicker of life in his eyes. But there was nothing. Just an expressionless face that was gradually becoming drained of color.

At some point during all of this, my supervisor appeared. He was a boyish forty-something named Dr. Jang, who had been tending to patients on a different floor. He was pudgy—one of the few doctors I met who could be described as overweight—and we exchanged a brief grunt of an introduction as I continued to pump away on Masterson's chest.

Every few minutes, just when I thought my arms were going to give out, Jang would nudge me aside and take over compressions. During those moments, as I stood behind him trying to catch my breath, I wondered what role nitric oxide had played in all of this. What was happening inside Masterson's body? And how long were we going to attempt to revive him? I'd never seen a team go beyond thirty minutes. But this guy was young and had a wife and two kids at home. How could we ever stop CPR? As I stood hunched over, with hands on my knees, I thought, *Don't let him die. Don't let this fucking guy die.*

Over the course of the year, I'd developed a belief that if I had touched a patient—if our flesh had made even slight contact—that person was my professional responsibility. This admittedly unusual view of the doctor-patient relationship had started sometime after my interaction with the drug mule, when I reflected on how absent I'd been during my exchange with her. That was me at my worst, a doctor just going through the motions, unmoved by the plight of a frightened young woman. That was not the physician I wanted to be. It wasn't the *person* I wanted to be. Once my palms had slammed into Dan Masterson's chest, I considered him mine. My patient. My responsibility. My problem.

Standing upright and straightening myself out, I again heard the voice of the ER doctor at the foot of the stretcher. "We have been performing CPR for twenty-two minutes. During that time the patient has remained pulseless. He has received three rounds of epinephrine and . . ."

I felt a tap on the shoulder and was instructed to resume chest compressions. More sweat fell as an IV was inserted into Masterson's groin and dozens of medications were administered. At one point, perhaps twenty-five minutes into the resuscitation, there was a brief blip on the cardiac monitor, possibly representing ventricular fibrillation. It was a good sign, potentially a sign of life, and we were all instructed to stand back as Dan Masterson was shocked with 120 joules of electricity. But it did nothing. There was no pulse and the monitor showed a flat line.

The flicker of hope had given us reason to press on, but as the minutes ticked by, one intervention after another failed. I found myself inadvertently holding my breath as each new medication was given. As I prepared to step back in and resume compressions, Dr. Jang cleared his throat and asked, "Does anyone object to calling it?"

I froze. We had performed CPR for nearly twice as long as I'd ever seen it done, but still, I didn't expect to stop. Dan Masterson was my patient, my first solo patient. On tomorrow morning's rounds, I was responsible for presenting every patient who'd been wheeled in to the ICU on my shift, and now I'd have to get up and say that we couldn't save him. I imagined the attending ICU doctors exchanging glances as I fumbled through an explanation of why we had failed. I imagined the whispers: *Does McCarthy know what he's doing?* I didn't want it to end like this. Dan Masterson had too much at stake.

There's always someone in the crowd who wants to keep going. I looked around for that person, but no one spoke. That someone was me. *Let's shock him again,* I wanted to say. *Let's shock him ten more times if we have to.* But I knew that wasn't the answer. You don't shock someone with a flat line on the monitor and no pulse. You need a fibrillating heart to use a defibrillator.

"Are we sure?" I asked. My eyes scanned the room, looking for someone to speak up. I felt for a pulse one last time. Nothing.

"Does anyone object?" Jang asked again. Every head gently shook from left to right, except mine. I knew they were right, but I didn't want to formally acknowledge it. I didn't want to accept that we had failed. "All right," Jang said, as he put his right hand on Dan Masterson's left foot, "time of death is ten twenty-one P.M."

My head dropped. My first patient was dead mere minutes after I had met him. I couldn't help him. What did this say about me as a doctor? Sure, I wasn't responsible for what had happened before he arrived—and I hadn't been the one running the arrest—but I hadn't been able to step in and revive him. I wanted to believe that repetition improved all of my clinical skills, every single one of them, from diagnosing pneumonia to cardiac resuscitation. But that wasn't the case.

So many parts of medicine are about process, and resuscitations are no exception. We were taught an algorithm for advanced cardiac life support. If no pulse, begin chest compressions. Get the patient on a heart monitor to see what's going on. Is there no heartbeat or a fibrillating heart? The best doctors move seamlessly through the algorithm, and the doctor who had run Dan Masterson's resuscitation had done a bang-up job, staying clear and focused during the longest effort I had been part of all year. And I had, I thought, been a perfect cog in the wheel. The whole resuscitation was a feat of well-orchestrated doctoring. The only problem was that the patient had died anyway.

It was an object lesson in the appalling limitations of medicine. I followed the proper technique—compress at least two inches, allow for full chest recoil—and the patient either lived or died. There is no art to it, no nuanced way to inject life into a lifeless body. Just mash on the chest and hope it works out. Looking at Dan Masterson's body, I made a fist with my left hand and smashed it into my right. What was the point in having all of this training and technology if we couldn't make it work?

I had seen so many patients brought back from the edge of death, so many saved when all hope was lost, but not this time. Baio had showed me what it was like to be special, to be a lifesaver, but tonight I was part of the losing team. And it made me wonder if I wasn't all that special without him. Or Don. Or Ashley. Or Moranis. Maybe I needed these more experienced doctors to effectively do my job. My arms and back ached, but my heart ached for Dan Masterson's family more. *Why did this happen?*

I stepped away from the body, and Dr. Jang put his arm around my sweaty shoulder. He could tell I was upset. "Did everything we could," he said.

"I know," I said, my eyes welling with tears. "Just fucking sucks. You know?" I couldn't quite explain why I was so emotional. What was it about this Dan Masterson? I had seen many patients die—at times it could be an everyday occurrence—and I rarely got choked up. The fiftieth death just doesn't jar you the way the first or second one does. But most of the people I saw die were elderly, or had been sick for a long time. I had participated in several failed resuscitations before this, but they had involved octogenarians who probably shouldn't have had to go through getting their ribs cracked at all. Dan Masterson was a young, good-looking guy who'd just walked in off the street and died. "I know," I said again. I wiped tears on my sleeve.

We looked back at Masterson's body as a nurse picked up the paper and plastic that had been chaotically strewn about the floor during the arrest, vial after vial of medication that had been administered in vain. There is something strange about acknowledging that life has exited a body. I don't believe in spirits fluttering up to the heavens or anything like that, but it did feel like something palpable had been taken away, extinguished and removed from the room as the pall of death slipped in. Soon, rigor mortis would set in and Dan Masterson's limbs would become stiff, his body cold. I focused for a moment on these biochemical processes to stave off the mental torment of his death and our failure.

"There's some paperwork that needs to be done," Jang said. He pulled a scut list from his white coat and put on a pair of tortoiseshell glasses. The man had clearly moved on to his next task. Was this me in a few years? I didn't want to know what it took to get there. "Do you know how to formally perform a postmortem exam?" he asked.

"Yeah."

"You also need to notify next of kin and request an autopsy," he said. "Have you done that before?"

"Yes." Death was a common, rarely unexpected part of my job, and a family member was usually nearby so the news could be broken in person. But I realized this next-of-kin conversation was going to be very different. I was about to call someone who didn't even know her husband was in the hospital. "I've never done it over the phone," I said. "Never called someone I haven't met." I tried to imagine how this might play out. Every scenario was horrible.

"You just gotta do it."

"Right."

"I know it's not helpful," Jang said more firmly, "but you just gotta do it."

As I tracked down Masterson's wife's name in the chart, my heart started to race. What would I say to her? These are the tasks—the heinous duties of being a doctor—that were never fully fleshed out in medical school, the awful moments you might never be comfortable with no matter how long you practice. We did occasionally practice delivering bad news—a new cancer diagnosis, or something equivalent—but nothing like this.

In that moment, as I slowly dialed her phone number, I wanted to disappear. I looked up at Jang after the final digit had been dialed. I felt like I was going to vomit. What should I say? What would I want to hear? If I received a call like this, I'd probably drop the phone and lose my fucking mind.

I heard the phone ring and took a deep breath. I still had no idea what I was going to say. Deliver the news fast, like ripping off a Band-Aid? Or slow, to give the woman time to wrap her brain around her new, horrific reality? The phone rang again, and I felt my pulse go even faster. I was now breathing rapidly and irregularly. Jang sat next to me, cracking his chubby knuckles.

After five rings, an answering machine picked up and I hung up the phone. "Do I leave a message?" I asked.

Jang shook his head. "Try again."

I called back, and a woman immediately answered the phone. "Mrs. Masterson?"

"Speaking."

"This is, ah, Dr. McCarthy from Columbia . . . from the Columbia University Medical Center. I'm calling about your husband."

"Is he there? What happened? Is he okay?" A television could be heard in the background. *You just gotta do it.*

"What's wrong with my husband?" she said quickly. "Tell me what's happening."

Much like I had done for her husband, I started to imagine what this woman might look like—confused, exhausted, frazzled—perhaps as a way of stalling. Was she holding one of her kids? What did her hair look like? "Tell me," she said again.

I looked at Jang, and he nodded. I turned away from him and bowed my head, staring down at my shoes, which were caked with Dan Masterson's blood. In the final instant, that last moment before I explained what had happened, my thoughts faded to black and I felt nothing. "Mrs. Masterson, your husband came to our emergency room earlier tonight."

"Oh, god," she whispered into the receiver. "Is he . . . Please tell me—"

"He had a cardiac arrest shortly after arrival and passed away ten minutes ago. We did everything we could. I am so sorry." I pushed the phone a few inches from my ear, but she didn't say anything. So I spoke to fill the void. "We attempted to resuscitate him for almost an hour, but our efforts were unsuccessful."

A muffled, bloodcurdling scream could now be heard in the background. For an unquantifiable unit of time I heard nothing but screams. I closed my eyes and fought off the urge to cry, to run away as ugly thoughts fluttered through my head. *I failed her. I failed her family. The world is an awful place. Her children will never know their father, and I played a role in that. Life is so fucked up.*

"Mrs. Masterson," I said eventually, "I want you to know that Dan, Mr. Masterson, is at the Allen Hospital."

"What is your name?" she asked softly.

"Matthew McCarthy," I said. "He . . . Mr. Masterson is at the Allen Hospital on Two Hundred Twentieth Street. Not the hospital on One Hundred Sixty-Eighth Street."

"And are you responsible?" she said more loudly. "Are you responsible for this?"

"I am one of the physicians who attempted to revive him, yes."

"I am coming in now," she said. "I am coming in now to find you, Dr. McCarthy." She hung up the phone, and I began to wait.

41

Jang patted me on the back and whispered, "Good job," as I hung up the phone and replayed the conversation in my head. Was she threatening me? It sure sounded like it. What would she do? Should I be worried? I tried to block her words out of my mind. I had work to do.

I sat down at a computer in the center of the ICU and prepared to write a death note—a medical-legal document explaining what had happened to Dan Masterson and what we had done about it—but I found myself unable to focus, not wanting to relive the failed resuscitation.

I turned away from the computer and leaned back in my chair. What would I say to Darby Masterson? And what about the hep C? Was I supposed to tell her about that, too? How much shit could I drop on one person? Your husband is dead, Darby, and oh by the way, I think he had hepatitis. I checked my pager and saw that while I was performing CPR, I'd missed nearly a dozen messages.

As I scrolled through the missed pages, I struggled to go back about my business as though nothing had happened. But that was what I needed to do. That hour with Dan Masterson was an hour where I had not been thinking about my other critically ill patients, and when I looked up from my pager, a line of nurses had formed to tell me what was happening around the unit. The Italian man had spiked another fever, and the Vietnamese woman had too much carbon dioxide in her blood. Oxygen was getting into her lungs, but carbon dioxide wasn't getting out, and that mismatch would soon cause her blood to become dangerously acidic.

I leapt out of my chair as a series of blood-gas equations flashed across my mind, like breaking news interrupting regularly scheduled programming. I needed to adjust both the frequency and amount of air being delivered by her ventilator, and quickly.

"Get some air," Jang said, intercepting me as I approached her room. "Take a breather."

I wasn't sure why he was still in the ICU; he had patients to see in other wings of the hospital. "I'm okay," I said.

He grinned and gently placed his hand on my chest. "I know you are. Just take five. Really. This is why I'm here."

"I'm fine. I promise you I'm fine."

He pointed at the exit. "Go."

I reluctantly stepped out of the unit, in search of food and a place to eat it, and noticed that my underarms were soaked with sweat. There were dark stains on my scrub pants—presumably blood or some other bodily fluid once belonging to Dan Masterson—and I still had a dozen more hours on call and untold obstacles to hurdle before I would be able to take a shower.

What did Mrs. Masterson mean by *I am coming in now to find you?* As I stood staring into the abyss of a vending machine several minutes later, my mind wandered across the hundreds of family members I had interacted with over the year. They were so unpredictable, so different. It was from them I learned that Carl Gladstone was a Yankees fan, that Denise Lundquist's best friend was her brother. Families provided invaluable windows into our patients' lives, transforming two-dimensional stories about chest pain into three-dimensional experiences for us to dissect and analyze as we went about our days. Peter Lundquist never left Denise's side, gently weeping as he watched her sleep. He prefaced every inquiry with *I don't want to bother you, Dr. McCarthy, but I have a tiny question about Denise.* Then he'd ask something that was not a tiny question, something like *Do you think we'll still be able to have children?* (They would.)

Families, in some ways, became our second set of patients. They needed time and attention, and if you failed to provide that, things could deteriorate quickly. Medicine is complicated and it is a skill to simplify things in a way that doesn't oversimplify, to accurately convey in plainspoken language what is actually happening inside another person's body. I made a conscious effort to do it, so it was irritating to see others doctors use medical jargon with families. Just talk like a normal person, I wanted to say. Pretend you're not a doctor. But for some, that simply wasn't possible.

Half an hour later, the nurse manager paged me that Dan Masterson's next of kin had arrived and had asked for me by name at the front desk. I passed Dr. Jang as I reentered the ICU—he was being called away to the emergency room—and as I sat down at a computer and waited for Darby Masterson to arrive, her voice began playing on a continuous loop in my head: *I am coming in now to find you, Dr. McCarthy. You. The one responsible.*

What if she had a gun? There was no metal detector at the front desk, just a drowsy security guard. And if she used it, would she even be guilty of anything? Wasn't this a heat-of-the-moment thing? *A doctor told me my husband was dead, Your Honor, and I went temporarily insane. I just started firing and now I throw myself at the mercy of the court.*

When Darby Masterson entered the intensive care unit, a trio of nurses met her at the door. I eyeballed her from a distance—about twenty feet away on the other side of the unit—and quickly discovered she wasn't quite what I had imagined. She was tall with very pale skin and had the soft paunch of a new mother. Long, dark black hair fell to her mid-back. She wore blue jeans, a dark blue sweatshirt, and gray tennis shoes. She did not look like a woman about to commit a violent act; she looked more like a victim, which she was.

As the nurses guided her into the room where her husband's body had been placed, we did not make eye contact. The room was closed off with a curtain, and the nurses stepped outside to give her privacy. I stared at the partition, trying to imagine what was happening on the other side and what I would say to her. Not long after she entered the room, I could hear the wails—the same sounds she'd made on the phone when I told her what had happened—but they were an octave lower now. I took a few steps back, as though the added distance might give her more privacy.

As the minutes ticked by, I tried to busy myself with other work—adjusting ventilators, writing notes, entering orders—but I couldn't focus. I kept waiting for Darby Masterson to emerge from her husband's room, but she never did. Hearing her unending sobs through the curtain, I knew this was not a woman who planned to attack me; this was a devastated widow who was here to grieve. And she deserved some semblance of an explanation, even if it was incomplete. I had to go in there; I had to talk with her. But given the amount of work that lay ahead of me, it couldn't be on her schedule. I needed to get this over with, and soon.

I could feel the nurses watching me as I slowly made my way across the unit toward Masterson's room. *You just gotta do it.* There was no way around this. It felt like I was about to do something very bad, as though my slow steps reflected inner turmoil. My mind wanted one thing—to enter the room—but my body wanted something else. When I was a few feet from the curtain, I announced myself and asked if I could enter. A faint voice said I could.

I opened the curtains to find Darby Masterson weeping at her husband's side. "I'm sorry to interrupt," I said, gently approaching the bed, "but I believe you were looking for me. I'm Dr. McCarthy." She stood up and turned away from her husband's body. She ran her hands through her dark hair and walked toward me. We stood a few feet apart, two strangers inexplicably thrown together through catastrophe. It took everything I had not to run away from her. "I am so sorry," I said.

She lunged at me and I briefly flinched, but chose to stand my ground. There was no violence, of course. Mrs. Masterson threw her arms around me and gave me a hug. I closed my eyes as her wet cheek met my collarbone and our abdomens lightly touched. Again my eyes glazed with tears. "I just want someone here to know about my husband," she whispered. "That's all I want."

"We did everything we could. We're still sorting everything out. I am so sorry for your loss."

"I just want someone to know."

"Tell me . . . tell me about him."

She took a seat and cried for several minutes. I wiped my eyes on my scrubs sleeve as I sat next to her and tried to imagine what she was going through. I simply couldn't. I ached for a blanket or a towel to cover my pants, to hide her husband's blood splatter. "My husband," she said, as she wiped the tip of her nose with a tissue, "I loved him so much."

I nodded, still not sure what I should say. "What was he like?"

Darby smiled through the tears and looked over at him. "He was a weird guy." She let out a sound that could almost be described as a laugh, and I tried to match her facial expression. "He wasn't a people person, he wasn't someone with a lot of friends. He was just a quirky guy who made me smile. No matter what kind of day I had, I knew he'd make me laugh when I got home."

"Sounds like a wonderful man." I wondered what tense I should use. Was it cruel to use the past tense, or simply accurate? "I wish I'd known him."

"He could also be moody," she said. "Lock himself in a room and surf the Internet for hours. Probably do it for days if I didn't stop him." I bowed my head and thought of Dan stumbling on nitric oxide therapy, reading the testimonials, ordering the package, hiding it away, and somehow inhaling the stuff into his body. This funny, moody guy had a secret, and I still wasn't sure if it was my job to reveal it. "I just don't understand," she said. "How could this happen?"

I looked at her and asked, "What do you know about your husband's medical conditions?"

She shook her head. "He was a pretty healthy guy."

"And did he take any medications?"

"Not that I know of. Maybe a multivitamin or something."

I paused, and tried to summon the wisdom to handle this properly. On the one hand, she deserved to know everything. On the other, I hadn't seen documentation that he actually had hep C or any other disease. It was something that had been told to me by another doctor; something that Dan Masterson said about himself, but he didn't arrive with any medical records to prove it. What if he hadn't used nitric oxide? What if he didn't have hepatitis? "Your husband lost consciousness shortly after he arrived in our emergency room. We still don't know why, but it appears he was using an alternative medicine to treat a medical condition. An infection. We weren't able to test him for it before—"

Her face went blank. "An infection?"

"Yes."

"What infection? What alternative medicine?" She shook her head. "What are you talking about?"

"He mentioned something to a doctor in the ER about nitric oxide therapy."

"Nitric oxide?" She straightened her back and looked at the ceiling. "For what?"

This was it. Darby Masterson deserved the truth, but I wasn't certain what the truth was. "People are trying it for all sorts of things," I said. "I didn't get to speak with your husband and he didn't come with any medical records, so we don't know for sure. But you're going to need to get tested—"

Darby flinched. "Tested for what?" We both looked at the corpse, and I considered my words. "Tested for what, Dr. McCarthy?"

I didn't know what to say. "It would be irresponsible for me to speculate," I said, "but it would be irresponsible for us to ignore what he said in the emergency room."

"What did he say?" Her eyes narrowed slightly, bracing for my answer.

From what I understood, hep C was usually spread by sharing needles; I wasn't sure if it was sexually transmitted, too. "You're going to need to get tested for a number of things, mostly viral diseases. I really can't say much more than that. Not without more information."

She stood up, and I joined her. Standing over her husband, I said, "I'm going to make a list of things you need to get tested for. And if I find out any more information, I will give it to you. I promise you that. We're still piecing together what happened here tonight."

"I am just very confused right now." She took her husband's hand in hers and nodded. We both wiped tears from our eyes.

"I . . . I just want you to—"

"Do you think I could have another moment alone?" she asked. "With my husband? Can we talk about this stuff a little later?"

"Of course." I slowly backed away from the Mastersons and slipped around the curtain and out of the room.

42

We never figured out why Dan Masterson died shortly after walking in to the emergency room. But before she left the hospital, I handed Darby Masterson a list of diseases she needed to be tested for and I also gave her my cell phone number and told her to call me if she ever wanted to talk. I had a strange union with her—I wouldn't call it a bond—and felt vaguely responsible for making sure things turned out okay for her. I knew I would remember Darby Masterson's bloodcurdling screams the rest of my life and suspected she might remember me, the ghastly messenger, for just as long.

About ten days later, as I staggered toward the subway after a thirty-hour ICU shift at the Allen, Darby called to tell me that every test had come back negative, including hepatitis C. I didn't tell her all that I'd heard about her husband because it was largely unconfirmed. I never saw his test result, and he'd died before one had been done at our hospital. Instead, I asked her to follow up with the physician who'd been caring for her husband, the one who had his medical records and could give her real answers. I wasn't sure if it was the right way to handle the situation, but it was a tremendous relief knowing she wasn't infected.

The remainder of my stint at the Allen Hospital ultimately lived up to its billing. The nights were exhausting and difficult—the tears for Dan Masterson weren't the only ones I shed that month—and those four weeks in the ICU were a crucial part of my development as an autonomous physician. I felt like I had assimilated medical knowledge with technical skill, empathy with tact, and somewhere along the way, perhaps around week two, I finally stopped hearing voices. When I examined my patients, I no longer thought of Don or Baio or Ashley, because I didn't need to. I knew what to do when I encountered a new patient, and I didn't need to be reminded. And if something stumped me, I was able to seek help and find the answer. Finally, after nearly a year of being an apprentice, I felt like I was ready to supervise another, less experienced doctor.

At the end of the month at the Allen, I was contacted by Dr. Petrak—the one with the Lithuanian eyebrows who once said I was working under a microscope—who told me that he'd heard about a clever diagnosis I had made and wanted to celebrate over a cup of coffee. He was referring to the frail Italian man, the one with the unexplained fevers that had confused my team for days. After poring over his records, I had discovered that his primary care doctor had recently placed him on a new medication and that drug, rather than an infection, had induced a fever. I relayed a bit of the story over the phone—"when I stopped the drug, the fevers just went away!"—but told Petrak I'd explain the rest in person. He was delighted, and without saying it, I knew that the microscope had been switched off.

Intern year ultimately drew to a close on a swampy day in June, one that forced Ali to wear something resembling shorts for the first time all year. On the subway ride to work, he appeared to be wearing lederhosen and was raising money for a group called Boys for Tots, which, according to his artisanal business card, sought to connect underprivileged young men with overprivileged yuppies in need of a babysitter.

It was a strange feeling walking into the main hospital on that final morning, knowing it would be my last as an intern, my last with the benefit of a second-year supervisor, and my last as a guy who could be forced to go on a predawn Starbucks run. Internship had been all-consuming, and my concern for what was happening in the world had gradually diminished as I'd thrown myself deeper into my work. (I was only vaguely aware that we were in the grip of a global recession and that mysterious things called subprime mortgages had been responsible for it.) Medicine had become my life. Everything else, everything that was not a matter of life and death, was now secondary. In some ways I was like a piñata, my insides scooped out and replaced with something new—something special—while my exterior had grown accustomed to taking a beating.

This year of sleepless nights had taken its toll on me. I had more gray hair on my head, several extra pounds around my waist, and two new chins. My eyes were hollowed out, and I'd developed the disturbing trait of occasionally falling asleep in mid-sentence. I looked quite a bit like Axel did when I met him.

Scenes from the year flashed before my eyes as I glided through the hospital's lobby on that bright June morning: Learning that Carl Gladstone was back at home plotting out his summer curriculum; trashing my stash of condoms after my HIV test had come back negative; consuming more Frostys than was safe for any human. One of the highlights had been hearing that Peter and Denise Lundquist had walked out of the hospital together, holding hands. The only thing missing, of course, was a heart for Benny.

More than once I had made the *Wizard of Oz* comparison in his presence. He was the Tin Man, in need of a ticker, and I was the Scarecrow, in need of a brain. Or at least a better one. But as the year progressed, I'd largely stopped seeing my life through the lens of a camera; I'd stopped viewing my work as a movie, one in which I just happened to have a starring role. This was not *The Truman Show*. As I became more comfortable doing my job, I felt less like an actor, less like someone playing a part. Medicine was a job and I was now comfortable doing it. I didn't need a script to follow.

The terrifying, inspiring year at Columbia had filled my brain with all sorts of knowledge—medical information, certainly, but so much more—things I wouldn't fully be able to process for years. I was still trying to work out a reasonable work-life balance, and through that struggle I had come to view my job like a new family member, an unpredictable stepbrother whom I mostly adored but, on occasion, couldn't stand.

Donning my white coat on that final day in June, I thought about something Baio had said much earlier in the year. *Everyone breaks.* Had I broken? Possibly. Probably. But then what? He and I never discussed what came after that. I had probably broken many times over, but now I felt like I had been reassembled, delicately patched back together, like they tried to do with Humpty Dumpty. The cracks were evident— they would always be there—but I was whole again, just in a slightly different iteration. The patchwork had been done by those close to me—my colleagues, my family, my friends, my advisers—those who wanted me to succeed. Overall, I was in a good place, relieved that the sleep deprivation and mental anguish hadn't done more lasting damage. I had survived intern year at Columbia, and now, when I said, "Amazing things are happening here," I meant it.

Mostly.

Despite those first few bumpy months, it had been the right choice to ditch surgery, to say good-bye to Axel and McCabe and MGH and move to Manhattan. I wasn't meant to suture up lacerations or remove gallbladders; I was meant to do whatever the hell you'd call the extraordinary stuff we did at Columbia. Intern year had fundamentally changed me—it had altered the way I viewed the world and myself— and it was unquestionably the most fun I never wanted to have again.

Now that I could make decisions quickly and confidently, I had more time to empathize with my patients, to see things from their perspective. To explore what might otherwise go unsaid during a brief visit in the hospital or in my clinic. And after a year of abandoning myself to medicine, I could now answer Diego's question with confidence: I was looking out for my patients, not myself.

As I was skipping up to the second-floor cafeteria, my thoughts turned elsewhere, to a conversation I'd had with Petrak a few days earlier about the storm that was building in higher education. Powerful educators were now claiming that medical school could plausibly be reduced from four years to three. In broad strokes, the argument was that so much of medicine was learned on the job and that medical school debt was driving many of the top minds into other fields. It was a highly contentious topic, and I had mixed emotions about it.

I learned very little physiology or pharmacology from Jim O'Connell, but the life lessons I absorbed from him would stick with me the rest of my career. How does one objectively measure the value of something like that? Would I have had time to wander the streets of Boston with Jim if medical school had been crammed into three years instead of four? As I loaded a stack of pancakes onto my plate on that final day, I heard a voice call out my name.

"Matisyahu!" Mark said, as he strutted toward me. "We made it!"

"We did," I replied, with a touch of relief and a touch of regret. I wondered what emotions he was experiencing. Was Mark broken? If so, the goofy grin on his face did a nice job of concealing it. I really didn't know what was going on inside his head. He and I were work friends, but that was about it. Our schedules so rarely overlapped that most plans to grab a beer and get to know each other were inevitably canceled. And it was more often my fault than his.

"Coming to karaoke tonight, Matty?"

"Of course." Tonight the senior residents were covering the interns' overnight shifts; it would be the first time since that autumn retreat in the Palisades that all of the interns would have an evening free together.

"What's your karaoke jam?" he asked. "I'm going with Cher and/or Naughty by Nature, depending on time constraints." I raised an eyebrow. He dipped his hips and wagged an index finger at me. "I'm naughty by nature not 'cause I hate ya."

Mark was clearly not experiencing the same twinge of regret I was. In that moment, I wished that I knew more about him. More about all of my colleagues, really. I'd had substantive conversations with so few of them. Had Mark broken down in tears? Had he stuck himself with a patient's bloodied needle? Did he ever think about leaving medicine? I had no idea.

"I might fire up Journey," I said as we stepped out of the elevator. "Or maybe the Outfield." He shrugged; the band's name clearly didn't register. Perhaps it was a poor choice for karaoke. "You know, the one that goes, 'I don't wanna lose your love tonight.'" It was the tune playing in my head as Banderas had counseled me after my needle stick and it was the song Heather and I would one day walk out to at our wedding.

"Huh."

"I could also do the Goo Goo Dolls."

"Oh please, no!"

"I might have to," I said. "I'll blame it on the sake."

"Don't blame it on the sunshine," Mark sang in falsetto, "don't blame it on the moonlight . . . just blame it on the sake."

"Nice."

"Michael Jackson, nineteen seventy-eight."

"Very nice." I couldn't remember the last time I'd been in the presence of such unabashed intern joy. Maybe the year had been harder on him than I'd realized. Or maybe he was just a fun-loving goofball.

"Maybe your pod could do reverse Black Eyed Peas," he said. "I could see you as Fergie. Corset and fishnets." I wondered how much sake it would take to convince Lalitha to be will.i.am. "For the big finish I'm doing Celine," he said, putting his left hand on my forearm. "If I touch you like this . . ." He grabbed my left hand and put it on his chest. "And if you kiss me like that . . ." I pulled my hand away as a nurse glanced at us.

"You are a nut."

"I am, Matisyahu. I am! See you tonight, pal."

We quickly ate our food and parted ways. I was finishing the year on the general cardiology service, and Benny, battling a case of pneumonia, was one of my patients. I headed over to his room to check on him, but he wasn't there. Unlike Dre, however, I knew he couldn't have gone far.

I headed down a long hallway and found him in a communal area, holding court. Seated in a horseshoe around him were five middle-aged men and women, nodding and taking notes as he spoke. Benny looked like a doctor conducting rounds, and those surrounding him appeared to be patients, or family members of patients, presumably dealing with similar medical conditions. Some were probably on the transplant waiting list.

"The thing is," Benny said, "this isn't easy. And it's not something that is going to be cured like that." He snapped his fingers and a woman raised her hand.

"How do you know if you're retaining fluid? They told me to take an extra dose of Lasix if I have a salty meal, but sometimes I just can't tell."

"Great question," Benny said. "I weigh myself every day. If I'm up a few pounds, I take an extra dose of . . ." He looked at me and trailed off.

"I'll come back," I whispered. "Thirty minutes?"

"Cool," he said, smiling as he returned to the group. "Where was I?"

We reconvened in his drab, straw-colored room a short while later, and I took a seat on the edge of Benny's bed. The relative calm of the general cardiology floor was a far cry from the bells and whistles we had grown accustomed to in the cardiac care unit. "Should I call you Professor?" I asked. "Or Doctor?" I smiled and patted him on the back.

"Just trying to pay it forward."

"I think it's great."

"So, this is it," he said. "Last day, right? You made it through."

"I did. It was some crazy shit. And some pretty amazing shit."

"Proud of you, Matt."

I thought about delivering some vaguely prepared remarks. A few words I had been mulling over in my head for months that would sum up what Benny's presence in the hospital had meant to me and to others. I wanted to tell him about his reputation as the embodiment of courage and patience—a kind man who had been given a raw deal and rarely complained.

I wanted to say something we'd both remember. But I didn't. Instead I repeated that phrase that I had said so often to him—the words I tossed off to countless patients, colleagues, and, most frequently, to myself: "You're gonna get through this." But it meant something different here, something far more personal. I wasn't saying this just to say it; I was saying it because I needed to believe it. And I wanted him to believe it. I had accused others of having gilded personas, but in this case I was the one possibly putting a false gloss on something, trying to adorn a difficult situation with unwarranted optimism. But I needed to say it.

I recalled the day I'd bumped into Baio at the vending machine, in the aftermath of my needle stick, when he said, "You'll get through it." The words had meant something to me then, even after he'd conceded that he said that to everyone. I grinned at Benny and picked up one of his Babyface CDs. "A bunch of us are going to karaoke tonight. Maybe I should try this out. A little slow jam."

Benny shook his head. "I would pay to see that."

He turned on the television and methodically flipped through the channels, and I sighed. "Oh please, please not *Judge Judy*." I felt my pager buzz. "Listen," I said, "I gotta get to rounds. Last one as an intern. Gonna try not to go out with a bang."

"I'm sure I'll see you around," he said, extending a fist.

"No doubt."

Walking out of the room, I glanced at a ripe banana peel in his trash can and smiled. "Benny," I said as I closed the door, "you really are going to get through this."

Epilogue

A few weeks later I found myself back in the CCU, standing in front of Carl Gladstone's old hospital bed, doing my best Baio impression. I was now a second-year resident, and before me were four anxious, enthusiastic interns—a new pod—waiting for rounds to begin.

I had spent the final weeks of intern year dissecting my initial struggles and had come to the conclusion that early on, I simply hadn't had the capacity to fully immerse myself in my patients' realities. I was so busy trying to master the medicine—to listen for a murmur or a wheeze rather than a note of despair—that I'd missed out on crucial opportunities to intervene in my patients' lives.

In my primary care clinic, I spent much of the year trying to ensure that my patients had all of the right medications—at times in excess of twenty different pills—and neglected to ask if this was ever too much. I failed to notice the wrinkled brow or the look of distress as I handed someone two dozen prescriptions to fill. But as the year wore on, I developed the ability to think outside the diagnosis, beyond the *science* of medicine to the *art* of medicine. I discovered that there is so much more to being a doctor than ordering tests and dispensing medications. And there is no way to teach that. It simply takes time and repetition.

There had been no ceremony to mark my transition from intern to supervising resident; I'd just shown up one day with a new assignment, a new list of patients, and a new group of exuberant, unwrinkled understudies. I wanted to see how far I could push them.

"Okay, Frank," I said, pointing to a tall African-American man. "Twenty-four-year-old black girl is found unresponsive in her hospital bed. You're first on the scene. Go."

Frank squeezed his stethoscope before running his hands down his crisp new white coat. "Twenty-four, let's see . . . twenty-four . . . and you said it's a woman?"

"The clock is ticking, my friend. And you're stalling."

As my intern pondered the scenario, I turned to the group. "A wise man once said that when you arrive at an arrest, the first pulse you should take is your own." They scribbled down the pithy statement, and I whipped my stethoscope around my neck. "Last year," I went on with more than a hint of swagger, "my residents had a scoreboard. One column was for arrests, one for lives saved, and they actually had one for arrests called while pooping. I'm still waiting for—"

A voice from a speaker a few feet above my head screeched: *AR-REST STAT, SIX GARDEN SOUTH! ARREST STAT, SIX GARDEN SOUTH!*

A rotating schedule had predetermined that today, the day before my thirty-hour CCU shift, was my day to run any cardiac arrest that occurred within the friendly confines of Columbia University Medical Center. It was a day I'd been thinking about for months. Years, really. This was the first arrest where I was going to run the show. *Showtime.* I dropped my scut list and broke out in a sprint.

"Good luck!" Frank howled as I crashed through the CCU doors. "No pooping!"

I'd rehearsed this moment in my mind hundreds of times. I'd thought about it over dinner with friends, on the subway, at bars, on airplanes, in my bed. This responsibility, more than any other part of being a doctor, was what I fixated on. The stakes simply couldn't be higher.

I sprinted down the long hallway and up a flight of stairs, trying to stay calm. Or calm*ish*.

ABC, ABC

Time slowed down as objects from intern year passed me in slow motion. To my left was Dave's office, to my right the vending machine I'd abused after the initial feedback session. As I passed the elevator Dr. Chanel and I had taken in the aftermath of my needle stick, other physicians joined me in the all-out sprint to Six Garden South: Ashley, Lalitha, Mark, and Don. More followed behind them. It looked like a scene out of Pamplona, except we were the ones doing the chasing. When we arrived at the sixth floor, a nursing aide pointed down another hall and said, "Fourteen. Bed fourteen."

As I entered the room full of people, Baio's voice caromed into my head: *You have to take command of the room.*

"I'm Matt," I said forcefully, "and I'm the arrest resident." They were the words I'd said into a mirror hundreds of times, words that I hoped would establish my authority. A dozen heads turned in my direction, just as I had imagined, and I positioned myself at the foot of the bed. As I looked at the patient before me, an unconscious, middle-aged white woman, words were shouted in my direction.

"Ms. Cardiff, forty-seven-year-old with coronary artery disease . . ."

A stream of phrases continued at me like an additional stanza to Billy Joel's "We Didn't Start the Fire."

"Hepatitis C in 1993."

"Blood sugar 103 . . ."

"Deep vein thrombosis in 2006."

"Platelets 170."

"No pulse."

Those two words smacked me in the face. "Mark," I said, addressing my colleague at the head of the bed, "do we have an airway?"

He held up an index finger and said, "Yes."

"Is she breathing?" I asked, as calmly as possible.

He squeezed a bag of oxygen down into her throat and said, "Not on her own, but I got her."

A team of anesthesiologists arrived a moment later and inserted a breathing tube into her trachea. "Lalitha," I said, "does she have a pulse?"

My pod mate mashed down on the woman's groin. "No."

"Don," I said, "please start chest compressions." Don had already started chest compressions.

"Too many people," a nurse announced and shooed several medical students away.

I took a long breath and said to the nurse beside me, "Please give one round of epinephrine and one round of atropine." The medications were at my side a moment later and inside the woman's pale, thin arm a second after that. I watched as Don continued to crack ribs, paced to the beat of the Bee Gees, as defibrillator pads were slapped on the woman's chest and back.

The unconscious patient was exceedingly thin, like a skeleton wrapped in a tiny layer of flesh. Perhaps she had a chronic illness—cancer, tuberculosis, or cirrhosis—that robbed her of excess muscle and fat. But there was no time to think about that. I knew all eyes were fixed on me. Someone handed me the woman's morning lab results. All normal. "Do we have central access?" I asked.

"Almost," Lalitha said, brandishing a large needle toward the woman's groin. "Okay," she said, "got it."

"Epi and atropine are in," the nurse said.

I looked at the cardiac monitor. "Please hold compressions," I said, "and check for a pulse."

As Lalitha felt the groin for a femoral pulse, we waited. And waited. Eyes slowly turned to me.

"I see a blip!" a voice near the door shouted. "We got a pulse!"

Lalitha looked at me and shook her head. No pulse.

"Definitely a pulse on the monitor!" said another.

They were making the same mistake I'd made a year earlier in the CCU. A blip on a monitor was not the same thing as a pulse. In fact, the two could be entirely unrelated, but that was a subtle point not always appreciated by physicians-in-training. "No," I said firmly. "We do not have a pulse. Resume chest compressions."

There were faint whispers in the periphery—students and residents discussing my decision—as the team went back to work. More epinephrine was infused into the woman as a new intern named Claire tried in vain to acquire arterial blood from the patient's wrist, so we would know how acidic the lifeless body had become. She readjusted the needle time and again, trying to find the tiny artery, as beads of sweat formed on her forehead. Claire knew everyone in the room was now looking at her, watching her fail over and over.

She stepped back from the body, closed her eyes, and took a deep breath. *I've been there*, I wanted to say, *just stick with it*. Claire's freshly pressed green scrubs now had a small, rapidly expanding sweat stain under each armpit. A moment later, she was edged out of the way by Mark, who took the needle from her and immediately hit the artery. The syringe quickly filled up with blood, and he sent it off to the lab seconds later as the sweaty intern looked on, crestfallen.

I scanned the patient's chart for possible clues. Why had this woman suddenly lost her pulse? Nothing jumped out at me. And I didn't have time to give the chart a close read. I felt the glare of the room, knowing that they were waiting for me to make a decision, relying on me to figure out what to do. I felt the urge to say something, to dole out more instructions, but there was nothing to say. We were following protocol and it just wasn't working.

"Please hold compressions," I said a minute later, "and feel for a pulse." The room fell silent as Lalitha explored the woman's groin. Several minutes had elapsed since we had begun the resuscitation, and as with a missing child, hope diminished with every passing moment. I gritted my teeth as I awaited Lalitha's call. Two dozen people watched me watch her.

Please have a fucking pulse, please.

I imagined saying the words "Does anyone object to stopping the resuscitation?" as I waited. What if someone objected, would I have to listen? Did it have to be unanimous? I'd never seen someone object. This would certainly be an unfortunate time to be confronted with that—

"We have a pulse," Lalitha said softly, "we definitely have a pulse."

"We have a pulse," I repeated. *Did everyone hear that? We have a pulse!* "We need a blood pressure," I said calmly, as Don strapped the blue cuff around the woman's arm. "We need a pressure," I said again.

"One ten over sixty," Don said. "Yesssss!"

"We have a bed in the ICU," a voice behind me whispered. It was Ashley. "They're ready. Let's move her."

"Let's move her," I said loudly, "ICU. Now. Lalitha, keep a hand on that pulse. Let me know if you lose it."

She nodded. The crowd parted, and we wheeled the patient in the direction of the ICU. As we emerged from the room, I saw Baio, standing in a corner watching the events. He winked at me. At least I think he winked at me.

——●——

In mid-May, second- and third-year residents and a smattering of faculty gathered to celebrate the end of the academic year. It was a boozy affair, a chance to send off the graduating residents, roast the chief residents (I sent in more than a few suggestions), and thank our professors. We also doled out awards. Some were serious—Most Likely to Win the Nobel Prize, Best in a Cardiac Arrest—and some were lighthearted—Best Looking in Scrubs and Cutest Couple. As dinner was served and drinks mixed, faces of finalists, whom we'd all voted for, flashed on a large screen. It was an outrageously fun night and one of the few times we collectively socialized. It was perhaps the only time that we saw one another in cocktail attire and certainly the only time we might have caught the Badass doing a shot.

It was the end of my second year of residency, and seated at my table were Lalitha, Meghan, Ariel, Ashley, Heather, and Mark. "Can I refresh anyone's cocktail?" I asked the group.

I was decked out in the only suit I owned—the one I'd worn to my medical school and residency interviews—and the same one I'd pulled out of the closet a month earlier for my infectious disease fellowship interviews. I had briefly toyed with the idea of becoming a critical care doctor, responsible for running an intensive care unit, but I kept coming back to those moments on the ninth floor of the hospital, with Dre and Dr. Chanel and the needle stick. I'd had a glimpse of the world of HIV medicine, a small insight into what these men and women were dealing with, and I wanted more. I also wanted to understand why bacteria and fungi were ravaging Benny's body, attacking his lungs, his liver, and his sinuses. "Drinks?" I asked again.

"The table politely declines," Ariel said, taking a gulp of Chardonnay.

It was a thrill to see my pod mates in makeup and cocktail dresses, and I was starting to get a bit tipsy; for once, we looked like the ones who belonged in *Us Weekly*. They were the reason I had survived the slog of residency, but I wouldn't fully understand that until I'd left them and had to practice on my own, as an attending at a different hospital in a different part of Manhattan.

In addition to being slightly drunk, I experienced a touch of melancholy as I looked around the ornate, wainscoted room. There were so many people who I never got to work with, never got to know. They all seemed so much happier right now, outside of the hospital. Glancing around, I realized that I had never met Dr. Sothscott after that fateful phone call in the CCU so many months ago. Was it possible I'd misheard his name? I never did find it in the hospital directory. Had it been someone using a pseudonym so he could freely blast me? I scanned the crowd and stopped at Mark, who was buoyantly wagging his index finger at me.

"Belieeeeve," he sang to our table, "when I say . . . I . . . want it that way!"

I was staring down at my dark and stormy, contemplating the need to use the restroom, when Heather grabbed my elbow and smiled.

"I'm fine," I said.

She pointed at the screen and nudged me; my face had just appeared as one of the five finalists for Best in a Cardiac Arrest.

A wave of pride washed over me. I had worked hard to demonstrate that I could calmly command a chaotic room, to not only appear calm but actually feel that way. To squelch the oh-shit-this-is-happening sensation when an arrest was called and act like bringing someone back to life was a routine part of my day. But knowing other doctors had voted on this was particularly special. "It's an honor," I said, to no one in particular, "just to be nominated." The words were intended to sound like a joke, but I meant them.

Meghan stuck her index finger in her mouth and pretended to gag. When Baio's face flashed on the screen as one of the other finalists, I looked over at him, but he was in mid-conversation with a pair of Lithuanian eyebrows. And next to them was Banderas. *Was Banderas wearing a blouse?*

A chief resident read out our names and then narrowed the group down to a final two: Baio and me. I looked over again, but he still wasn't paying attention to the ceremony. How was he not paying attention to this? I was anxious and excited, probably more nervous now than during an actual cardiac arrest. I was also weirded out. How was my name mentioned in the same breath as Baio's? "What will America decide?" I said, sotto voce, as I picked at my entrée. "It's like the People's Choice Awards."

"Best in a cardiac arrest," the chief resident announced, "is Matt McCarthy."

Of all the things that could've crossed my mind in that moment, my first thought was of uncooked spaghetti—the sensation I'd experienced when I first performed CPR on that ninety-five-year-old woman in the CCU on my first night on call. It was inconceivable that the physicians at Columbia thought I deserved this over Baio, the man who'd shown me how to do CPR. The guy who'd taught me just about everything I knew. He was the best doctor I'd ever worked with, someone who seemingly knew how to handle any situation. If I had a medical question, I'd turn to him. If someone dropped dead in this room, I'd want *him* leading the resuscitation.

Heather gave me a kiss on the cheek and whispered, "Congratulations," as Lalitha, Meghan, and Ariel gave me high fives.

"Ladies," I said, trying to hide my slight embarrassment, "if any of you would like an advanced tutorial on the art of cardiac resuscitation, we can arrange private lessons. You'll find that my rates are competitive with—"

"Oh, barf," Lalitha said. "Please stop. No acceptance speech."

"Shut it down," Heather said.

Maybe I'd grown; maybe I *was* better than Baio. The learning curve was steep, and perhaps I'd just barely nudged past him. I looked around the room to relish the moment, to catch the cheers of encouragement from my colleagues. Dr. Petrak gave me a thumbs-up, and Mark was whistling wildly through his fingers. I smiled, kissed Heather, and gave Mark a fist pound. Taking another long sip of the dark and stormy—a sip that was bound to nudge me from tipsy to intoxicated—I felt someone come up behind me, squeeze my neck, and whisper, "You're welcome."

— ◦ —

A year later, as I was on the verge of graduating from Columbia's residency training program it happened. Standing in a conference room—the same room where Dave had demonstrated the proper way to perform phlebotomy after my needle stick—I felt my pager vibrate. Before me was a gifted young medical student named Christopher, and I was again channeling Baio. I had completely shed the paranoid urgency and trepidation of intern year and was now dressed casually— khakis and a button-down—because I was on a research elective and

Petrak had asked me to spend my spare moments teaching medical students. "Forty-seven-year-old woman is found unresponsive," I said, recalling the first arrest I'd run on my own. "Go."

"Okay, okay," Christopher said, twirling his curly dark hair. "Okay, what else?"

"That's it."

Staring at this young man, I thought of all of the experiences that lay before him: the arrests, the tears, the grief, the joy, the rapture. The strange enchantments of medicine. I also couldn't help but reminisce on all that I had seen and done in my three years at Columbia. Remarkably, I used the reply-all button only once during residency, after our besotted awards dinner, when I wrote, "Heather is pregnant. Just kidding," and shared a link to a Vampire Weekend song called "I Think Ur A Contra."

My pager buzzed again. I halted the role-playing with Christopher and glanced down at the four words on my pager's tiny screen: HE GOT THE HEART.

"Holy fuck," I said. "Let's go." I grabbed Christopher by the shirt-sleeve and tugged him out of the room with me. "Holy shit, c'mon!"

Sprinting down a flight of stairs to the cardiothoracic intensive care unit, Christopher must've thought we were on our way to an actual cardiac arrest. I nearly trampled an Orthodox Jewish couple and quickly started scanning the beds in the unit. *No, nope, not him, not him, nope, no, no, YES!*

The page wasn't tagged, meaning I had no idea who'd sent it, but scores of doctors knew that I was close with Benny and that I'd want to know if anything happened to him, good or bad. I sidled up to the team of surgeons and anesthesiologists standing in front of his room. Benny was attached to a ventilator and had a dozen tubes going into his arms, like I'd seen him so many times before. As we approached, a surgical intern was presenting his case to a team of transplant doctors, ". . . year-old man postoperative day zero status postcardiac transplantation. Currently sedated and stable on—"

"Do you guys know this patient's story?" I asked, butting into their horseshoe to address the medical team. "Do you know anything about this guy Benny Santos?"

Like Darby Masterson, I just wanted someone to know. Anyone. The young physicians stared at me blankly, blinking quickly, before consulting their scut lists. But there was nothing on their papers to indicate how special Benny was. To them, he was probably just another transplant patient. My eyes were met with blank stares. We stood in silence until I let out a celebratory yelp. "He got the fucking heart!"

One of the surgeons wrinkled his brow. "Are you from social work?"

I slipped on a gown and gloves and prepared to enter Benny's room. "No," I said, fighting back a smile. "I'm not from social work."

"Respiratory therapist?" another asked.

Without the scrubs or white coat, I didn't quite look like a doctor. I was just some enthusiastic, slightly unhinged guy in loafers who didn't mind interrupting their rounds. I nodded at Benny and said, "I've known this guy a long time." I was about to elaborate, about to provide an anecdote that offered a glimpse into the life of this remarkable man, but I caught myself. How could I possibly explain what Benny had been through or what that struggle meant to me? I turned away from the team of doctors and took a few steps closer to him—his body once again attached to a ventilator, but this time, finally, with a new heart—and I smiled. The stories could wait. "Take good care of this guy," I said softly. "I'm not his doctor anymore. Now . . . just a friend."

I picked up a remote control sitting on the nightstand next to Benny's bed, turned on the television, and started flipping through the channels until I found *Judge Judy*.

Acknowledgments

This book exists because of one person: my editor, Kevin Doughten. ~~Good~~ Great guy.

Heather, my girl, you've endured far too many moments when, staring into your eyes, my thoughts were a thousand miles away, reliving a cardiac arrest. You are the best person I know, and every day that I wake up next to you is a good one.

Acknowledgments would not be complete without thanking my family: my mother, Belinda, who introduced me to *Talking Heads;* my father, Bernie, who really is holding out hope that I become a dermatologist; and my sister, Megan. *Who loves you, baby?*

I am fortunate to be surrounded by a wildly talented group of friends—Rach, Charlie, Ben, and John—and by thoughtful people who worked so hard on this book: Claire Potter, Lauren Kuhn, Danielle Crabtree, Jessica Miele, and Sarah Kwak, to name just a few. Scott Waxman, a wonderful agent and friend, thank you for your continued support and encouragement.

I also want to acknowledge the men and women who work at Columbia making the world a better, more dignified place. And to the patients who have trusted us, thank you.

ABOUT THE AUTHOR

MATT McCARTHY is an assistant professor of medicine at Weill Cornell Medical College and is on staff at New York–Presbyterian Hospital. His work has appeared in *Sports Illustrated, Slate, The New England Journal of Medicine,* and *Deadspin,* where he writes the Medspin column. His first book, *Odd Man Out,* was a *New York Times* bestseller.